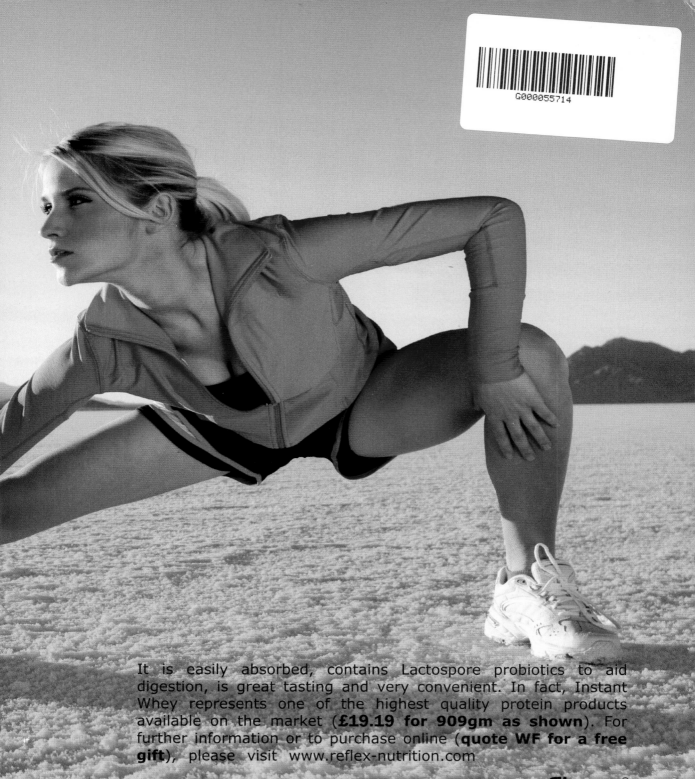

It is easily absorbed, contains Lactospore probiotics to aid digestion, is great tasting and very convenient. In fact, Instant Whey represents one of the highest quality protein products available on the market (**£19.19 for 909gm as shown**). For further information or to purchase online (**quote WF for a free gift**), please visit www.reflex-nutrition.com

FULL MONEY BACK GUARANTEE

reflex®
Tomorrow's Nutrition Today™

women's fitness magazine

BODY SHAPE WORKOUT

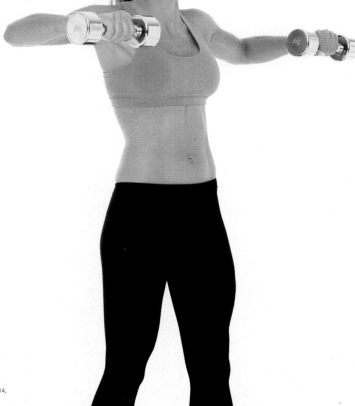

Cover clothing: Casall Sports Bra, £39.99, King's Road Sporting Club, www.krsc.co.uk, 020 7589 5418, Interlock Running Shorts, £16, American Apparel, www.americanapparel.co.uk
Workout clothing: Hi Tech Sports Bra, One Step Ahead @ King's Road Sporting Club, £29.99, www.krsc.co.uk, 020 7589 5418, ProForm Tights, £27.99, www.proformfitness.co.uk, 0845 177 0514, ASICS Gel-Kayano 16 Trainers, £120, www.asics.co.uk
Exercise equipment: Reebok, www.johnlewis.com and The Physical Company, www.physicalcompany.co.uk, 01494 769 222

Welcome to the Women's Fitness Bodyshape Workout

Women come in all different shapes and sizes, from apple and pear to hourglass and boyish. Each shape is equally beautiful, but you can make the most of yours by doing certain exercises, eating a particular diet and using a cardio routine tailored to your specific shape.

Understanding and working with your bodyshape will make your health and fitness gains so much easier. Different shapes have a tendency to store fat in different places, but by working with your body and adopting a healthy diet, combined with cardio and toning exercises, you can change your bodyfat composition.

The easy-to-use tailored cardio, food and toning plans in this book will help you make the most of your bodyshape in just four weeks. Not only will you learn what works for you and your body, so you can incorporate it into your lifestyle in the future, but you'll also be inspired by the fitness goals you can achieve, regardless of the level you're starting from.

So, whatever your shape, this book will not only help you accentuate all your favourite parts, but will also create new ones, giving you a gorgeously toned body in just four weeks.

Learning what makes your bodyshape tick will allow you to work with it and really make the most of it – so what are you waiting for?

Enjoy the book, and your bodyshape!

Joanna Knight, Editor

For more training tips, workouts and the latest fitness news, visit our website at www.womensfitness.co.uk

Editor **Joanna Knight**
Sub-Editors **Karen Staddon, Lucy Cheek, Felicity Cloake**
Art Director **Matt Reynolds**
Senior Designer **Stephen Beerling**
Writers **Jeff Archer, Sue Hay, Anne-Marie Lategan**
Photography **Eddie Macdonald (cover and workouts), istockphoto.com**
Cover model **Anel, www.motmodels.co.uk**
Workout models **Carolina Narte Pereira , W Athletic, www.wathletic.com**

**INTERACTIVE
PUBLISHING PLC**
3rd Floor, 207 Old Street
London
EC1V 9NR
Tel: 020 7608 6300

Contents

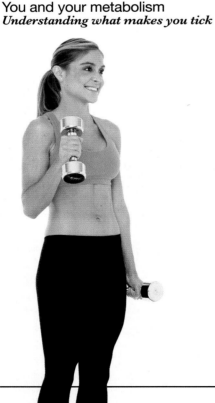

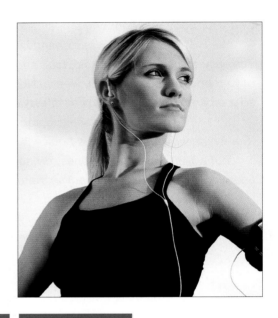

7

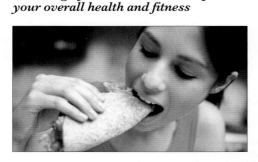

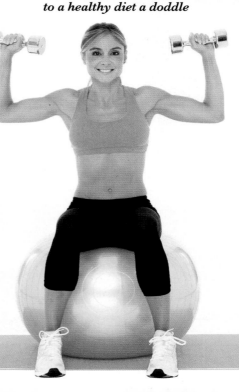

How to use this book

USING THE BODYSHAPE WORKOUT COULDN'T BE SIMPLER – JUST IDENTIFY YOUR BODYSHAPE THEN FOLLOW OUR TAILOR-MADE PLANS!

↘Your bodyshape

First things first, find out what your bodyshape is – if you're unsure, use the simple guide on page ten to diagnose yourself. As each bodyshape has its own characteristics, read up on yours and learn where you store bodyfat and why, discover the best type of exercise for you and find out how to make the most of your shape.

Results in four weeks

This is a four-week regime and includes toning exercises, cardio plans and tailored food plans for each bodyshape. Combine the cardio workouts with a variety of exercises for best results. Each bodyshape has a tailored four-week cardio plan, with beginner, intermediate and advanced options, so whatever your fitness level, you can really make the most of the plan for your particular shape.

Over 80 exercises

There are over 80 exercises that you can mix and match to keep challenging your body. Certain bodyshapes will want to work some areas more than others; for example, pears will work more on their bottom and legs, while boyish shapes should focus on their upper body and waist. Simply pick at least one exercise for each body part (arms, chest and shoulders, waist and stomach, core, back, bottom, legs and balance) and then get started!

How to design your workout

For each exercise, body types are listed in order of priority. If body type apple is listed first, then this means that it is very important for apples to include more than one exercise from this category in their workout in order to maximise their results. Follow the sets and reps at the beginning of each section according to your fitness level: beginner, intermediate or advanced. You can use different levels for different sections; if beginners' legs get too

8

'A new fitness routine is enhanced by a great diet; one that offers you enough energy to work out, and to repair and restore your muscles'

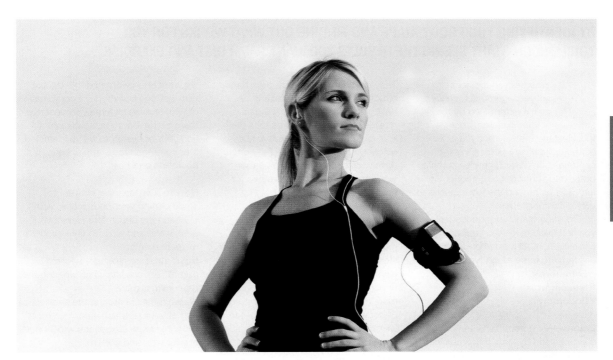

easy, move on to intermediate but keep your arm workout at the beginner level. For each of the weight-training workouts, pick eight to ten exercises depending on the amount of time available. Design two to three workouts to maximise results and stop boredom.

Easy-to-use food plans
A new fitness routine is enhanced by a great diet; one that offers you enough energy to work out, and to repair and restore your muscles. The food plans are specifically designed to be easy to use, featuring plenty of store cupboard ingredients and quick recipes, so eating healthily doesn't become a time-consuming chore. Simply mix and match a breakfast, lunch and dinner from the individual bodyshape plans.

The best shape of your life!
The combination of specific food, cardio and exercise plans will accentuate your bodyshape, boost your energy levels and get you in the best shape of your life, in just four weeks. Don't forget, though, if you are about to embark on a new fitness regime and you have been inactive for any period of time, be sure to check that it is safe to do so with your doctor. Most importantly, however, remember to enjoy yourself and work with your bodyshape, and in no time you'll have your best body ever!

Which bodyshape are you?

BY IDENTIFYING YOUR BODYSHAPE AND FINDING OUT WHAT WORKS FOR YOU, YOU'LL SOON START SEEING THE RESULTS YOU WANT FROM DIET AND EXERCISE

Your bodyshape is not something you can choose, as it's determined by the structure of your skeleton, your muscles and the way bodyfat is distributed on your body. Over the centuries our view of the ideal female bodyshape has changed frequently, and women around the world aspire to very different shapes.

To understand your bodyshape, you first need to look at your body's classification. All human bodies can be divided into three rough types:

• **Ectomorph**
• **Mesomorph**
• **Endomorph**

Ectomorph: Ectomorphs are characterised by long, thin limbs with light bones, small joints and small muscles. Because of their small muscles, ectomorphs are usually not very strong. They have low levels of fat and are often referred to as tall and slim. They have a fast metabolic rate and find it easy to lose weight, but very hard to put on muscle weight. Ectomorphs are usually an hourglass or boy shape.

Mesomorph: Mesomorphs usually have very athletic-looking bodies.

They are characterised by large bone structure and a solid torso, and usually have good posture. They will gain muscle very quickly, but despite their lean look, they will pick bodyfat up quicker than ectomorphs. They often have wide shoulders and a narrow waist and are classified as a pear or hourglass shape.

Endomorph: Endomorphs are characterised by short limbs and a round, soft body. Most of their fat storage is around the waistline. They have a large bone structure and the upper parts of their limbs are usually more developed than the lower parts. Endomorphs find it very hard to lose weight and are usually hourglass, apple or pear-shaped.

Very often women don't identify with just one body type; a combination of two, or even all three, will describe them better. So, to make it easier to find your bodyshape, we've identified four common types: apple, pear, hourglass and boy.

How to identify your shape
To determine your bodyshape, you will need the circumferences of your bust, waist and hips. To take accurate measurements:
Bust: measure around the fullest part of your breasts when wearing a properly fitted bra.
Waist: measure around the smallest part of your stomach area.
Hips: measure around the widest part of your hips and bottom.

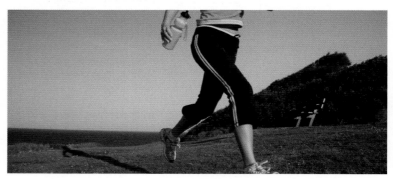

did you know?

Since the 1950s, women's waistlines have expanded by six inches. They are also taller with bigger busts and hips.

(Source: H. McCormack)

Hourglass
If you have a big bust, small waist and a generous bottom, then you are an HOURGLASS shape, which is the most voluptuous of body types. However, you have a tendency to gain weight all over. To find out more, go to page 12.

Boy
If you are slim with a straight-up-and-down shape and no noticeable curves at your waist, hips or bottom, then you are a BOY shape and probably find it very difficult to put on weight anywhere. To find out more, go to page 14.

Apple
If you have a big bust, waist and tummy, you are an APPLE shape, as you have a tendency to gain weight around your middle. Bodyfat is stored deep under the skin, which can lead to health problems if not monitored. To find out more, go to page 16.

Pear
If you are small on top but have relatively big hips, then you are a PEAR shape as you tend to gain extra weight around the hips, bottom and thigh area. Bodyfat is stored just under the skin. To find out more, go to page 18.

Waist-to-hip ratio (WHR)
Your waist-to-hip ratio (WHR) is your waist measurement divided by your hip measurement. This figure, although not the most accurate, has been used by doctors to determine your risk of developing heart disease because it indicates if a person is prone to store bodyfat around the waist or not. Research has also found that the WHR is an indication of attractiveness in most cultures across the world (David Buss, *The Evolution Of Desire*, 2003). A WHR of 0.7 was found to be the most attractive by European men compared to 0.6 for China and 0.9 in Africa. A value of 0.7 means that your waist circumference is 70 per cent of your hips' circumference.

Changing your bodyshape
You may be born with a specific body type, but there are numerous factors that can temporarily or permanently change your shape.
• **Age:** Ageing causes the level of female hormones to lower, which leads to an increase in bodyfat storage, especially around the waistline.
• **Diet:** Different body types will respond differently to certain diets and foods and, interestingly, each bodyshape can often be attracted to particular calorie-laden foods. So knowing which foods to avoid can help you to achieve your weight-loss goals and improve your appearance.
• **Exercise:** Don't train harder, train smarter! If you slave away in the gym and are not seeing the results in the areas that you want to, you are doing something wrong! Exercise does work, but if you are not doing the correct exercise combination for your body type you are not going to experience the results you want, however hard you try.

11

Hourglass

EVERYTHING HOURGLASS SHAPES SHOULD KNOW ABOUT THEIR BODY AND HOW TO KEEP IT IN TIP-TOP CONDITION

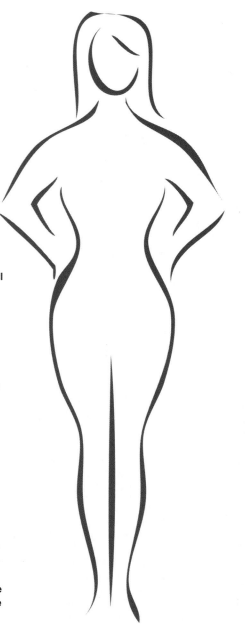

What is the hourglass bodyshape?

For centuries the hourglass shape has been the most desired bodyshape for men and women. The hourglass figure has perfect proportions between the chest and hip measurements, with a smaller waistline. A true hourglass body will have about six inches difference between the chest and waist.

What happens when hourglass shapes gain weight?

Hourglass women usually have high metabolic rates, which means they don't put on weight very easily. When hourglass women do gain weight it tends to be evenly spread all over their bodies, thus making it less noticeable. This lucky body type is also the least likely to develop cellulite. If they do get it, the cellulite will be concentrated around their bottom area and on the back of their thighs.

What type of exercise should hourglass shapes do?

Hourglass shapes tend to tone up quickly and therefore should use light weights with higher repetitions. Their toning programme should include equal amounts of upper and lower-body exercise to maintain their shape. Cardio exercise is also important to control weight-gain. Cardio exercise that works both the upper and lower body will be more beneficial to hourglass shapes as it will help to keep their body in proportion.

Which celebrities have hourglass bodyshapes?

Hollywood legends such as Marilyn Monroe and Jayne Mansfield were regarded as having perfect hourglass figures in the Fifties. Now the shape is back in fashion among today's stars who prefer having a voluptuous frame to being a size zero. Holly Willoughby and Nigella Lawson both have the hourglass look down to a tee.

What else should hourglass bodyshapes know?

Researchers at Harvard University in the US found that curvy women have higher female hormone levels than other women, which boosts their fertility and makes them more likely to conceive. It was suggested this could be the reason why the hourglass figure was traditionally viewed by men as the ideal female bodyshape.

12

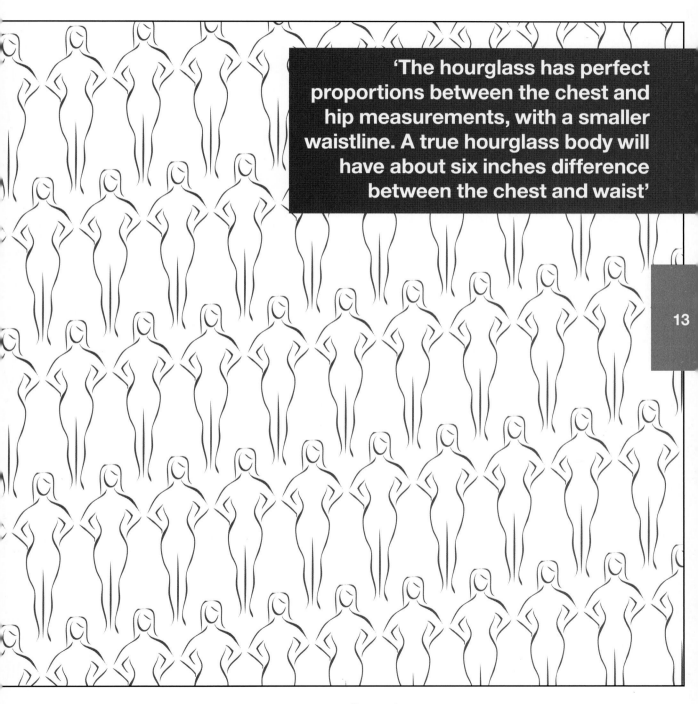

'The hourglass has perfect proportions between the chest and hip measurements, with a smaller waistline. A true hourglass body will have about six inches difference between the chest and waist'

13

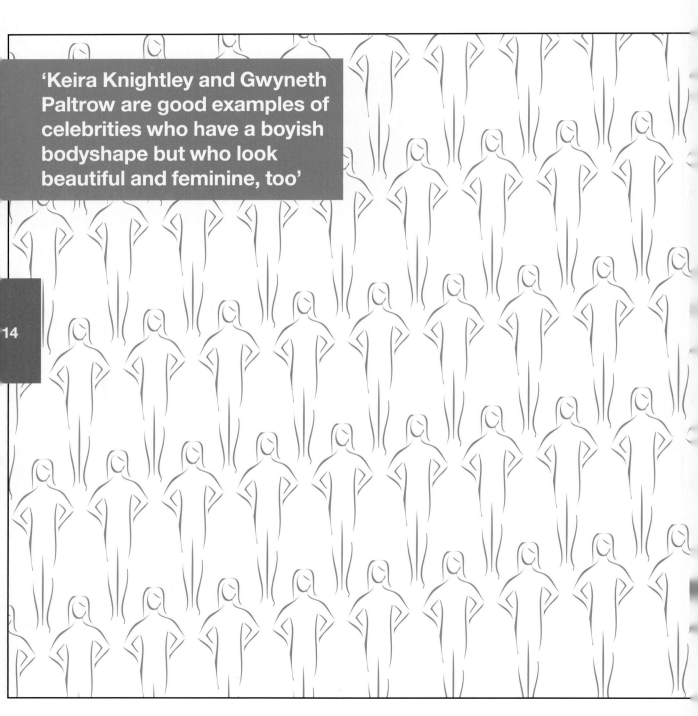

'Keira Knightley and Gwyneth Paltrow are good examples of celebrities who have a boyish bodyshape but who look beautiful and feminine, too'

14

Boy

EVERYTHING BOY SHAPES SHOULD KNOW ABOUT THEIR BODY AND HOW TO LOOK AFTER IT

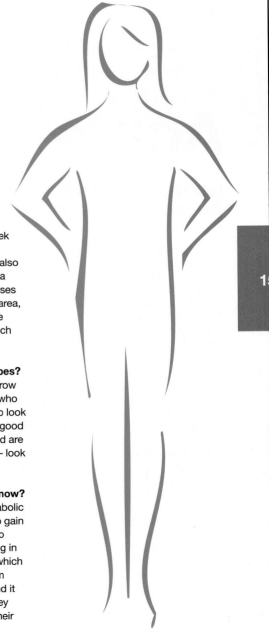

What is the boy bodyshape?

Boy shapes tend to have wide, muscular shoulders and no discernible waistline, a boyish, flat bum and straight legs. They usually have good muscle definition in their arms and legs but there are no significant differences between the chest, waist and hip measurements, giving a straight-up-and-down look.

What happens when boy shapes gain weight?

Boy shapes look very lean, but when they gain weight they add fat around their waist, stomach and bottom. If boy shapes pick up too much fat weight they can easily change into the apple shape, which can have serious health implications including diabetes and heart disease.

What type of exercise should boy shapes do?

Toning exercises will help boy shapes to gain more curves. In most cases boy shapes have toned, lean arms and legs; however, it is important to add stomach, core and waist exercises at least three to four times per week to shape and develop a waistline. Doing plenty of cardio exercise is also important to control bodyfat. Use a variety of cardio and toning exercises to prevent bulking up in a certain area, and keep the weights light and the repetitions high to prevent too much muscle gain.

Which celebrities have boy shapes?

Keira Knightley and Gwyneth Paltrow are good examples of celebrities who have a boyish bodyshape but who look beautiful and feminine, too. Most good athletes have muscular bodies and are usually classified as boy-shaped – look at Paula Radcliffe.

What else should boy shapes know?

Boy shapes have a very fast metabolic rate and don't have a tendency to gain weight, but they can easily fall into the trap of eating junk food lacking in essential vitamins and minerals, which is not beneficial for their long-term health. Boy shapes will usually find it easy to pick up muscles when they train, which in turn will increase their metabolic rate even more.

15

16

Apple

EVERYTHING APPLE SHAPES SHOULD KNOW ABOUT THEIR BODY AND HOW TO KEEP IT IN GREAT WORKING ORDER

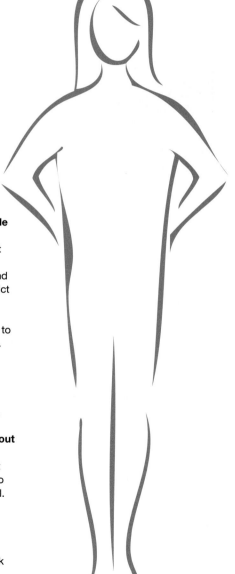

What is the apple bodyshape?

Apple shapes have a round figure, although this does not always mean they are carrying extra weight. All their fat is distributed around their waist, chest and upper back area, and they generally have large breasts, small bottoms and slim legs. Their waist measurement will often be larger than their chest and hip measurement, and cellulite is very common. Many celebrities described as an hourglass shape are actually more like apples.

What happens when apple shapes gain weight?

Being apple-shaped makes you more likely to gain weight, and also puts you at a higher risk of Type 2 diabetes and heart disease. Apple-shaped women have a slow metabolism, which makes it easy to gain weight but hard to lose it again. Fat cells around the stomach produce chemicals that can damage the body's insulin system, so this makes it all the more important that you follow a healthy diet and lifestyle.

What type of exercise should apple shapes do?

Exercising using a combined weight and cardiovascular programme is important to reduce your bodyfat and increase your metabolic rate. Be strict with your programme: never train in your comfort zone. If your workout gets too easy, increase the intensity to ensure results and prevent plateaus.

Which celebrities have apple shapes?

Drew Barrymore, Lorraine Kelly and Catherine Zeta-Jones are all apples.

What else should apples know about their shape?

High stress levels can also cause fat deposits around your waist thanks to the influence of the hormone cortisol. Exercises alone will not be enough to prevent obesity or reduce your risk factors; diet will also play a very important role in controlling your weight and hormone levels, so check out our food plans for apple shapes, starting on page 150.

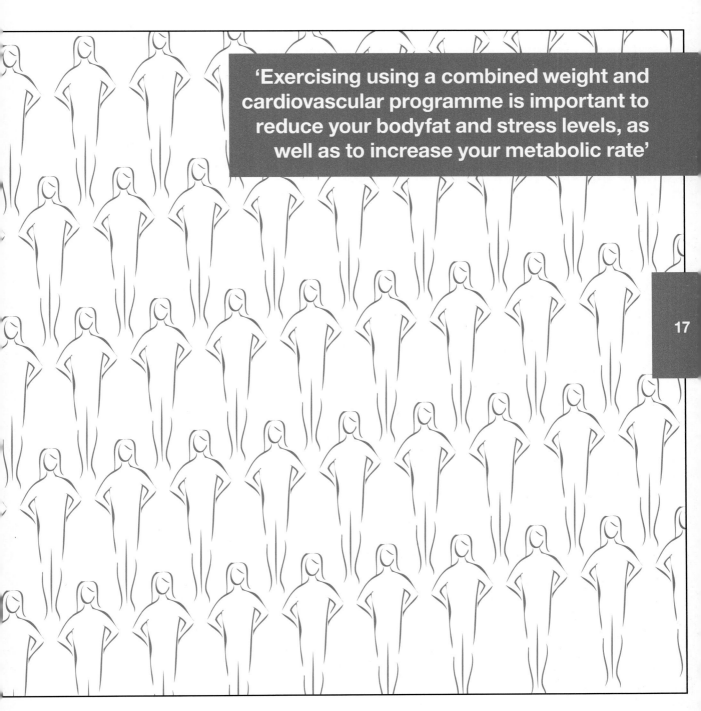

'Exercising using a combined weight and cardiovascular programme is important to reduce your bodyfat and stress levels, as well as to increase your metabolic rate'

17

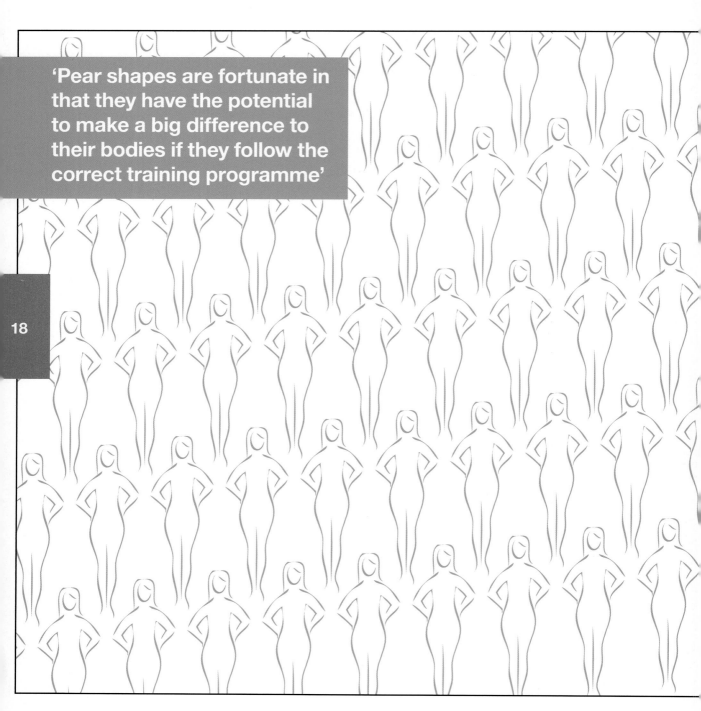

'Pear shapes are fortunate in that they have the potential to make a big difference to their bodies if they follow the correct training programme'

18

Pear

EVERYTHING PEAR SHAPES SHOULD KNOW ABOUT THEIR BODY AND HOW TO GET THE BEST FROM IT

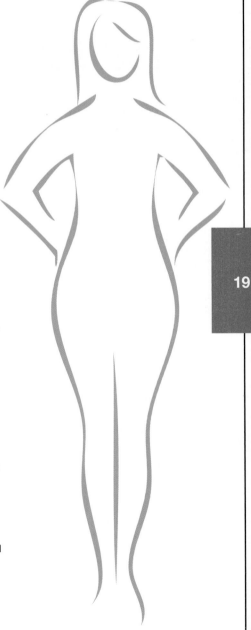

What is the pear bodyshape?
The curvaceous pear usually has a small upper body with lean arms and a narrow waist. All the bodyfat is distributed around the lower stomach, hips, thighs and bottom, and the hip measurement will be bigger than the waist and chest. However, this isn't always a bad thing: wide hips are a traditional sign of fertility, and are considered extremely desirable in many cultures around the world.

What happens when pear shapes gain weight?
Pears are more prone to cellulite than other shapes due to the concentration of fat around their hips. They have, however, less chance of developing medical problems like heart disease. Pear shapes are fortunate in that they have the potential to make a big difference to their bodies if they follow the correct training programme.

What type of exercise should pear shapes do?
The classic pear-shaped woman has a well-defined waistline and an enviably flat tummy, so most of their training programme should be focused on their bottom and legs. Cardio exercise will help get rid of excess bodyfat, but it's the toning exercises that will help pear shapes fit comfortably into skinny jeans. Choose cardio exercises (e.g. swimming or cross-trainer) that involve the whole body, rather than legs only, to prevent your legs from bulking.

Which celebrities have pear shapes?
Jennifer Lopez, Kate Winslet and Coleen Rooney are great examples of celebrities who have made the most of their shape without having to resort to extreme crash diets.

What else should pears know about their shape?
Research shows that women with a hip measurement of 40 inches (size 14) or more appear to have some level of protection against heart disease that is absent in slimmer people. That's because hip fat contains a natural anti-inflammatory called adiponectin, which prevents arteries swelling up and becoming blocked. Storing fat around the hips also has far fewer health risks than storing fat around the waist, although, as with all bodyshapes, it's important to maintain a weight that's healthy for your height.

19

For best results

TO REALLY MAKE THE BODYSHAPE WORKOUT WORK FOR YOU, JUST FOLLOW THESE SIMPLE RULES…

When starting any fitness plan, you have to really want to do it in order to get results. So, first of all, consider what your goal is – it could be to complete a forthcoming sporting event, a personal resolution to be your healthiest ever, or to improve your self-esteem by becoming more body confident.

Once you've found your motivation and decided to embark on this plan, these simple steps will help you achieve your health and fitness gains safely and enjoyably!

1. Diagnose your body type. Doing so will allow you to learn more about your bodyshape's tendencies and preferences, so you can work with your body, not against it.

2. Establish which cardio level you're at: beginner, intermediate or advanced. Pushing yourself above your level will reduce your fitness gains and leave you feeling de-motivated, whereas working within your level will ensure your body responds well to the training, and will give you the confidence to move to the next level when you are ready.

3. The 80-plus exercises in this book will tone your entire body. Certain bodyshapes will need to focus on some areas more than others, so at the beginning of each section, we've explained which bodyshape will benefit most from working this part; for example, boyish shapes will benefit from including waist exercises in their toning programme.

4. For best results:
For beginners, combine cardio exercise with 15 to 20 minutes of toning moves between three and four times a week. Pick a selection of one, two or three exercises for each body part, adding more if your shape requires it.

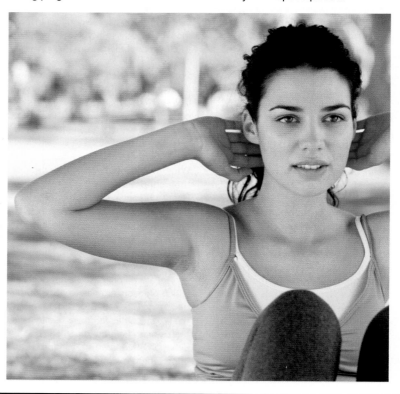

20

'Consider what your goal is – it could be to complete a forthcoming sporting event, a personal resolution to be your healthiest ever, or to improve your self-esteem by becoming more body confident'

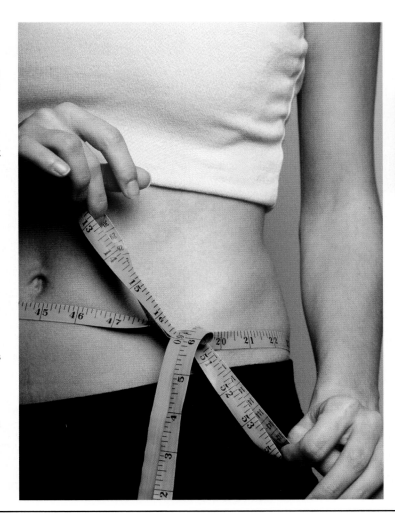

For intermediates, combine cardio exercise with 20 to 30 minutes of toning exercises between three and four times a week. Pick a selection of one, two or three exercises for each body part, adding more if your shape requires it.

For advanced, combine cardio exercise with 30 to 40 minutes of toning exercises between three and four times a week. Pick a selection of one, two or three exercises for each body part, adding more if your shape requires it.

5. Be sure to warm up and cool down before any exercise, and remember to stretch your major muscles after exercise (see page 38 for tips).

6. Combine your cardio and training plans with the four-week food plan (which starts on page 137). Each bodyshape craves certain foods, and knowing what your body wants and responds to will help you achieve maximum health and fitness gains and avoid unnecessary weight-gain.

7. Finally, enjoy it. To really get the most out of a new routine you have to want to do it, so make sure that the cardio options and toning exercises you choose are fun, even if they are hard. And if there are some you really don't like, do them first and get them out the way. The ones you prefer rarely have the best results!

Motivation tips

GETTING ACTIVE MAY SEEM LIKE A DAUNTING TASK, BUT KEEP YOUR END GOAL IN MIND AND IT WILL BE MUCH EASIER THAN YOU THINK

There's no doubt that the hardest part of any exercise plan is getting started. Once you're up and running, experiencing the mental benefits of a more active lifestyle and seeing the physical changes to your body, pushing yourself to maximise your progress can still sometimes be a challenge – but it isn't nearly as daunting as that very first step of the journey.

For many people, it's the thought that there's no guarantee of results that makes getting started so difficult. It's not surprising really. The idea of making all that effort for no reward doesn't sound too motivating does it? It's like going to the shops, handing over your hard-earned cash, and getting nothing back in return.

The reason most people worry about the results they'll get is because they judge by past experience, but just because you didn't get the results you were looking for then, doesn't mean things will be the same now.

Don't give up!

Often, people don't experience the results they want because they embark upon the wrong programme for their objectives, or they aren't flexible enough with their approach. The most common attitude is to try something for a short time, and if it works, great, but if it doesn't, then to give up. A

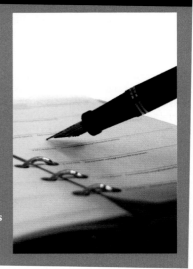

5 top tips for getting started

- **Begin now, don't delay. The more you procrastinate, the harder it is to get going.**
- **Keep your end goal in mind at all times. Thinking about the results you want will motivate you far more than worrying about the steps you need to take in order to achieve these results.**
- **Get support from others.**
- **Plan your exercise schedule and stick to it.**
- **Plan some (healthy!) rewards to enjoy when you achieve your results.**

more effective way of doing things is to consider that, if you aren't getting the specific results you want with your training programme, you need to modify it by tackling things from a slightly different direction. The thing to avoid at all costs is simply giving up.

This is particularly relevant when you are training for your bodyshape. Not all fitness plans produce the same results for different people with different shapes, but you must

persevere and experiment and try a variety of programmes and approaches until you can piece together the routine that works for you, and that gets you consistent results both now and in the long-term.

Find what works for you

Don't for one moment think that the bodyshape you have now is the shape you'll have forever. If you want to make changes, you can. All you need to do

22

'Pick a start date and begin with any exercise you like – if you find something you enjoy, it won't feel like a chore and you'll keep up the routine'

is pick a starting date and begin with any exercise you like. The key phrase here is 'exercise you like', because if you find something you enjoy doing, it won't feel like a chore and you're more likely to keep up a routine. In turn, sticking to this routine will guarantee that you get the results you're looking for. The speed at which this happens

depends on you and how quick you are to modify your routine to develop the techniques that work for your bodyshape, and drop the parts of your training programme that you consider will be less effective in helping to achieve the bodyshape you desire.

Obviously, you have to be realistic about how dramatically you can alter

your basic bodyshape, but everyone can enhance their natural shape by doing the right exercise and following the food plan that works for them. The main thing is to enjoy your bodyshape, work with it and make the most of every opportunity to get active, eat well, optimise your health and your fitness, and feel great every single day.

23

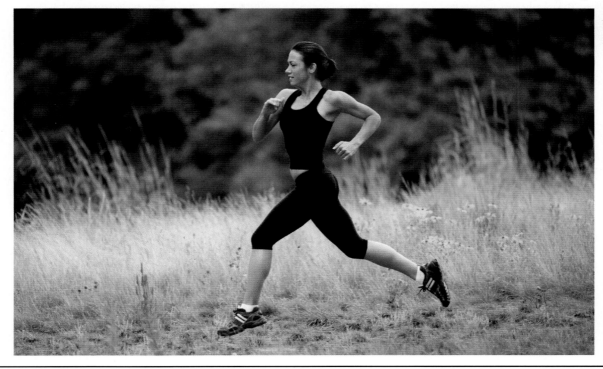

You and your metabolism

UNDERSTANDING YOUR METABOLISM IS THE KEY TO KNOWING YOUR BODY AND HOW IT WORKS

We all need to generate energy to survive, and this energy comes from the food we eat. Within our bodies, a series of chemical processes regulate all of our systems. These processes are known collectively as the metabolism.

The metabolism controls the various functions and reactions that keep our bodies running efficiently, including the digestion of food and nutrients, the elimination of waste products, respiration, circulation of the blood, regulation of body temperature, contraction of muscles and the function of the brain and nerves.

Our basal metabolic rate (BMR) is the speed at which our system operates while at rest. The amount of energy released at this point is sufficient to maintain all our essential body requirements, such as the heart, lung, brain and nervous system.

How's your metabolism running?
The speed at which your metabolism runs is relevant when it comes to

24

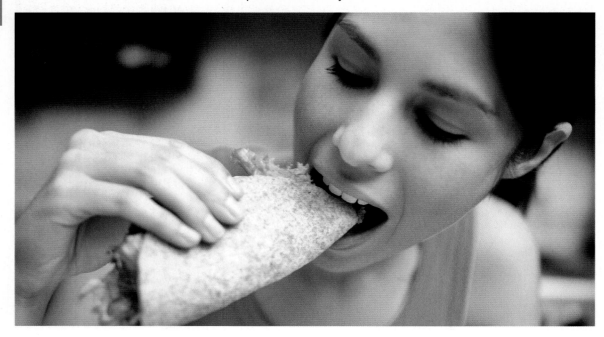

'Because strength training encourages the growth of lean muscle tissue, your metabolism will begin to run faster between workouts as well as during them'

thinking about bodyshape because if you consume more energy than you need to cover the requirements of your basal metabolic rate, the excess will be stored as bodyfat and could have a dramatic impact on your shape. Therefore, if your metabolism is slow you'll put on weight more easily. On the other hand, if your metabolism is running quickly, it will be much easier to burn calories and stay in shape. If you know someone who seems to be able to eat what they want without ever putting on a pound, chances are, they've got a fast metabolism.

As we age, our metabolism naturally slows, and, if we make no adjustments to our lifestyle, this may lead to a change in bodyshape.

How to boost your metabolism
Fortunately, it is possible to boost your metabolism at any age. The most important step for achieving this is to eat healthily and regularly. The process of digesting food creates heat and boosts your metabolism. Eat the right foods, including plenty of fresh fruit and vegetables, wholemeal carbohydrates, low-fat protein and essential fats (in the right quantities) and you'll find that your metabolism runs quickly and efficiently. Eat too

much of the wrong food, or deprive yourself of food, and you'll find that your metabolism will slow down.

Another way to boost your metabolism is with exercise, including both cardiovascular exercise and strength-training workouts. A simple way to understand how this works is to imagine your metabolism is a volume control, and your basal metabolic rate is like having the volume set to one. Your metabolism is running, but running slowly. When you go for a run or a swim or a bike ride, you're boosting your metabolism temporarily up to level 4 or 5, depending on the intensity of your exercise, as the demand for energy to perform the exercise increases. When you stop the cardio exercise, your metabolism returns to level one.

By performing strength-training exercises, not only do you temporarily increase your metabolism for the duration of the exercise, but, because strength-training encourages growth of lean muscle tissue (which is very active and requires a lot of energy to maintain), your metabolism begins to run faster between workouts as well as during them. So, over time, your basal metabolic rate increases as you crank up the 'volume' on your metabolism.

5 top tips to boost your metabolism

• Pack as much activity as you can into every day.
• Stay hydrated to help your system run efficiently at all times.
• Eat regularly, starting with breakfast and then continuing with meals and healthy snacks throughout the day.
• Add some spicy food to your diet.
• Eat natural rather than processed foods, and chew everything thoroughly.

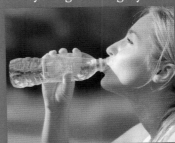

25

SPECIALISTS SAY A LITTLE RUSH OF ADRENALINE CAN CURE WHAT AILS YOU.

The Brooks Adrenaline™ GTS 9 - Our trustworthy 'Go To Shoe'

- Midfoot wrap, forefoot capture & progressive support loved by countless runners.

- Support combined with so much action in one shoe - a rare find.

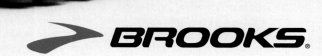

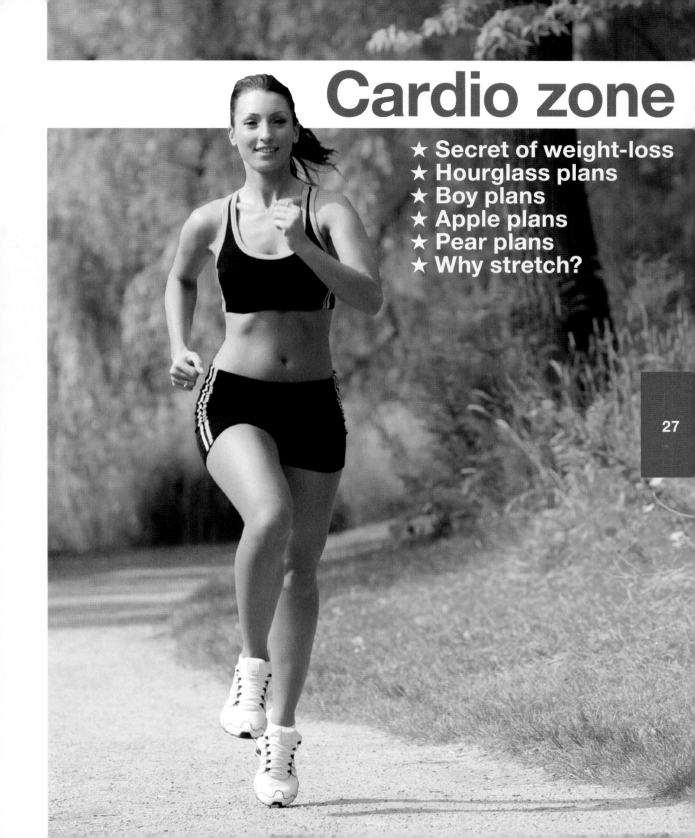

Cardio zone

★ **Secret of weight-loss**
★ **Hourglass plans**
★ **Boy plans**
★ **Apple plans**
★ **Pear plans**
★ **Why stretch?**

The secret of weight-loss

THE KEY TO TONING YOUR BODYSHAPE AND KEEPING IT THAT WAY IS A COMBINATION OF CARDIO AND WEIGHT-TRAINING

Whatever your bodyshape, the right mix of cardio and weight-training is vital for getting the results you want. Read on to find out why…

Get your heart rate up!

Cardio exercise is any activity that works your heart and lungs. If you're unsure whether an activity counts, ask yourself if you get out of breath while doing it – if the answer is yes then it's classified as cardio! Therefore brisk walking, jogging, running, swimming, aerobics, dancing and Spinning all fall into the cardio category.

Not only is cardio exercise the most effective way to burn calories when combined with a healthy diet, the workout it gives your heart also reduces the risk of developing high blood pressure, high cholesterol and heart disease. It evens boosts your energy levels and makes your skin glow.

Lift a little

Weight-training uses resistance in the form of free weights (dumbbells), fixed weights (gym machines) or your bodyweight (a press-up) to strengthen and tone your muscles. This in turn builds lean muscle tissue, which is vital for long-term weight-loss and controlling your bodyshape.

Our bodies require energy (calories) even to function at rest. The amount needed is known as your basal metabolic rate (BMR). As muscle cells require more energy to maintain than fat cells, the more lean muscle you have the higher your BMR will be and the more calories you'll burn, even when at rest. As you burn calories faster, your body will require more energy too – so don't reduce your calorie intake.

The main concern women have when it comes to weight-training is that they will bulk up, but lean muscle does not mean bulk. Bulky muscles come from intense periods of tough weight-training, whereas the exercises in this book will add subtle definition to your muscles – not bulk.

Calorie-burning cardio mixed with BMR-raising weight-training is the key to achieving and maintaining the bodyshape you want. Cardio workouts will help burn excess bodyfat and weight-training will tone your muscles – a winning combination!

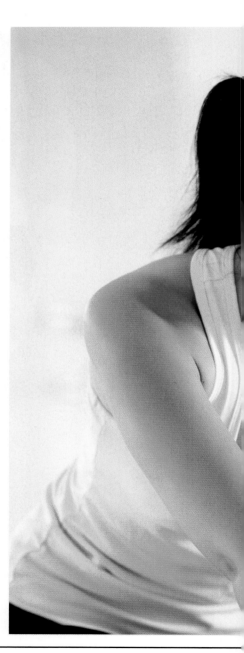

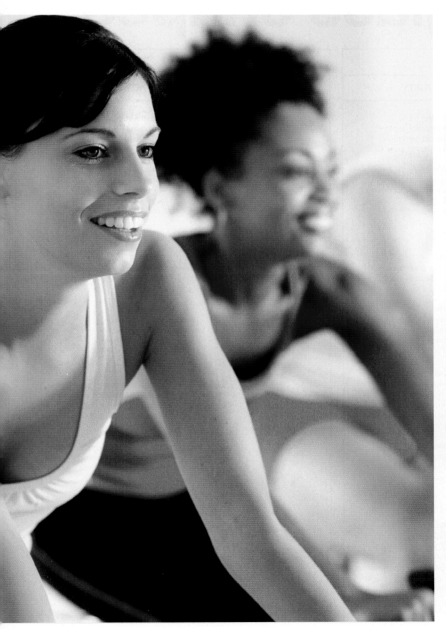

'Weight-training builds lean muscle tissue, which is a vital ingredient for long-term weight-loss and controlling your bodyshape'

Guidelines

Beginners (those who have been inactive for a period of time): aim for four sessions a week at an easy to moderate pace.

Intermediates (regular exercisers): aim for four sessions a week at a moderate to fast pace.

Advanced (you know who you are!): aim for four longer sessions a week at a moderate to fast pace.

Plans start on page 30.

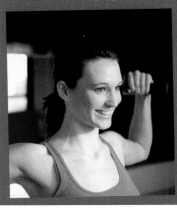

29

Hourglass shapes

WEEK 1	
DAY	**REPS & ACTIVITY**
MONDAY	**CROSS-TRAINER** **Beginner:** 20 minutes easy pace **Intermediate:** 30 minutes easy pace **Advanced:** 30 minutes moderate pace **ROWER** **Beginner:** 10 minutes easy pace **Intermediate:** 5 minutes easy pace, 5 minutes moderate pace **Advanced:** 10 minutes moderate pace
WEDNESDAY	**SKIPPING** **Beginner:** 10 minutes skipping / recovery **Intermediate:** 15 minutes skipping / recovery **Advanced:** 20 minutes skipping / recovery **RUNNING** **Beginner:** 15 minutes jogging **Intermediate:** 15 minutes running **Advanced:** 20 minutes running
FRIDAY	**CYCLING** **Beginner:** 10 minutes low resistance, fast RPM (revs per min) **Intermediate:** 15 minutes low resistance, fast RPM **Advanced:** 10 minutes low resistance, fast RPM, 5 minutes higher resistance, fast RPM **CROSS-TRAINER** **Beginner:** 20 minutes easy pace **Intermediate:** 30 minutes easy pace **Advanced:** 30 minutes moderate pace
SUNDAY	**CARDIO MEDLEY** **Beginner:** 10 minutes moderate-speed cycling, 10 minutes easy rowing, 10 minutes jogging **Intermediate:** 10 minutes moderate-speed cycling, 10 minutes moderate-pace rowing, 10 minutes running **Advanced:** 10 minutes fast cycling, 10 minutes fast rowing, 10 minutes fast running

WEEK 2	
DAY	**REPS & ACTIVITY**
MONDAY	**CROSS-TRAINER** **Beginner:** 20 minutes easy pace **Intermediate:** 30 minutes easy pace **Advanced:** 30 minutes moderate pace **ROWER** **Beginner:** 10 minutes easy pace **Intermediate:** 5 minutes easy pace, 5 minutes moderate pace **Advanced:** 10 minutes moderate pace
WEDNESDAY	**SKIPPING** **Beginner:** 10 minutes skipping / recovery **Intermediate:** 15 minutes skipping / recovery **Advanced:** 20 minutes skipping / recovery **RUNNING** **Beginner:** 15 minutes jogging **Intermediate:** 15 minutes running **Advanced:** 20 minutes running
FRIDAY	**CYCLING** **Beginner:** 10 minutes low resistance, fast RPM **Intermediate:** 15 minutes low resistance, fast RPM **Advanced:** 10 minutes low resistance, fast RPM, 5 minutes higher resistance, fast RPM **CROSS-TRAINER** **Beginner:** 20 minutes easy pace **Intermediate:** 30 minutes easy pace **Advanced:** 30 minutes moderate pace
SUNDAY	**CARDIO MEDLEY** **Beginner:** 10 minutes moderate-speed cycling, 10 minutes moderate-pace rowing, 10 minutes running **Intermediate:** 10 minutes moderate-speed cycling, 15 minutes moderate-pace rowing, 15 minutes running **Advanced:** 15 minutes fast cycling, 10 minutes fast rowing, 15 minutes fast running

WEEK 3

DAY	REPS & ACTIVITY
MONDAY	**CROSS-TRAINER** **Beginner:** 10 minutes easy pace, 10 minutes moderate pace **Intermediate:** 10 minutes easy pace, 15 minutes moderate pace **Advanced:** 10 minutes moderate pace, 10 minutes fast **ROWER** **Beginner:** 10 minutes moderate pace **Intermediate:** 5 minutes moderate pace, 5 minutes fast pace, 5 minutes moderate pace **Advanced:** 5 minutes moderate pace, 10 minutes fast
WEDNESDAY	**SKIPPING** **Beginner:** 10 minutes skipping **Intermediate:** 15 minutes skipping **Advanced:** 20 minutes skipping **RUNNING** **Beginner:** 10 minutes jogging **Intermediate:** 20 minutes running **Advanced:** 30 minutes running
FRIDAY	**CYCLING** **Beginner:** 15 minutes low resistance, fast RPM **Intermediate:** 20 minutes low resistance, fast RPM **Advanced:** 10 minutes low resistance, fast RPM, 10 minutes higher resistance, fast RPM **CROSS-TRAINER** **Beginner:** 10 minutes easy pace, 10 minutes moderate pace **Intermediate:** 10 minutes easy pace, 15 minutes moderate pace **Advanced:** 10 minutes moderate pace, 10 minutes fast pace
SUNDAY	**CARDIO MEDLEY** **Beginner:** 15 minutes moderate-speed cycling, 15 minutes moderate-pace rowing, 15 minutes running **Intermediate:** 20 minutes moderate-speed cycling, 20 minutes moderate-pace rowing, 20 minutes running **Advanced:** 20 minutes fast cycling, 20 minutes fast rowing, 20 minutes fast running

WEEK 4

DAY	REPS & ACTIVITY
MONDAY	**CROSS-TRAINER** **Beginner:** 10 minutes easy pace, 10 minutes moderate pace **Intermediate:** 10 minutes easy pace, 15 minutes moderate pace **Advanced:** 10 minutes moderate pace, 10 minutes fast **ROWER** **Beginner:** 10 minutes easy pace **Intermediate:** 5 minutes moderate pace, 5 minutes fast pace, 5 minutes moderate pace **Advanced:** 5 minutes moderate pace, 10 minutes fast
WEDNESDAY	**SKIPPING** **Beginner:** 10 minutes skipping **Intermediate:** 15 minutes skipping **Advanced:** 20 minutes skipping **RUNNING** **Beginner:** 10 minutes running **Intermediate:** 20 minutes running **Advanced:** 30 minutes running
FRIDAY	**CYCLING** **Beginner:** 15 minutes low resistance, fast RPM **Intermediate:** 20 minutes low resistance, fast RPM **Advanced:** 10 minutes low resistance, fast RPM, 10 minutes higher resistance, fast RPM **CROSS-TRAINER** **Beginner:** 10 minutes easy pace, 10 minutes moderate pace **Intermediate:** 10 minutes easy pace, 15 minutes moderate pace **Advanced:** 10 minutes moderate pace, 10 minutes fast pace
SUNDAY	**CARDIO MEDLEY** **Beginner:** 15 minutes moderate-speed cycling, 15 minutes moderate-pace rowing, 15 minutes running **Intermediate:** 20 minutes moderate-speed cycling, 20 minutes moderate-pace rowing, 20 minutes running **Advanced:** 20 minutes fast cycling, 20 minutes fast rowing, 20 minutes fast running

Boy shapes

WEEK 1

DAY	REPS & ACTIVITY
MONDAY	**WALKING / RUNNING** **Beginner:** 15 minutes incline walking **Intermediate:** 15 minutes incline walking / running **Advanced:** 10 minutes incline walking, 10 minutes incline running **STEPPER** **Beginner:** 10 minutes easy pace **Intermediate:** 10 minutes moderate pace **Advanced:** 10 minutes fast pace
WEDNESDAY	**ROWER** **Beginner:** 15 minutes easy pace **Intermediate:** 15 minutes moderate pace **Advanced:** 10 minutes moderate pace, 5 minutes fast pace **STEPPER** **Beginner:** 5 minutes easy pace, 5 minutes high resistance: long, slow steps **Intermediate:** 10 minutes high resistance: long, slow steps **Advanced:** 10 minutes fast pace, 5 minutes high resistance: long, slow steps
FRIDAY	**SWIMMING** **Beginner:** 20 minutes: 2 lengths fast, 4 lengths recovery **Intermediate:** 30 minutes: 2 lengths fast, 4 lengths recovery, and repeat for duration **Advanced:** 40 minutes: 2 lengths fast, 4 lengths recovery, and repeat for duration
SUNDAY	**WALKING / RUNNING** **Beginner:** 15 minutes incline walking **Intermediate:** 15 minutes incline walking / running **Advanced:** 10 minutes incline walking, 10 minutes incline running **WALKING / RUNNING** **Beginner:** 15 minutes easy pace **Intermediate:** 15 minutes moderate pace **Advanced:** 10 minutes moderate pace, 5 minutes fast pace

WEEK 2

DAY	REPS & ACTIVITY
MONDAY	**STEPPER** **Beginner:** 5 minutes easy pace, 5 minutes high resistance: long, slow steps **Intermediate:** 10 minutes high resistance: long, slow steps **Advanced:** 10 minutes fast pace, 5 minutes high resistance: long, slow steps **ROWER** **Beginner:** 5 minutes easy pace, 5 minutes high resistance, low RPM (revs per min) **Intermediate:** 10 minutes high resistance, low RPM **Advanced:** 10 minutes fast pace, 5 minutes high resistance, low RPM
WEDNESDAY	**WALKING / RUNNING** **Beginner:** 15 minutes incline walking **Intermediate:** 15 minutes incline walking / running **Advanced:** 10 minutes incline walking, 10 minutes incline running **RUNNING** **Beginner:** 15 minutes easy pace **Intermediate:** 15 minutes moderate pace **Advanced:** 10 minutes moderate pace, 5 minutes fast pace
FRIDAY	**SWIMMING** **Beginner:** 20 minutes: 2 lengths fast, 4 lengths recovery **Intermediate:** 30 minutes: 2 lengths fast, 4 lengths recovery, and repeat for duration **Advanced:** 40 minutes: 2 lengths fast, 4 lengths recovery, and repeat for duration
SUNDAY	**CARDIO MEDLEY** **Beginner:** 10 minutes moderate-resistance cycling, 10 minutes rowing, 10 minutes incline walking **Intermediate:** 10 minutes moderate-resistance cycling, 15 minutes rowing, 15 minutes incline running **Advanced:** 10 minutes moderate-resistance cycling, 15 minutes interval training on rower, 10 minutes fast-incline running, 5 minutes sprint-incline running

WEEK 3

DAY	REPS & ACTIVITY
MONDAY	**WALKING / RUNNING** **Beginner:** 10 minutes incline walking, 5 minutes incline running **Intermediate:** 10 minutes incline walking / running, 10 minutes incline running **Advanced:** 5 minutes incline walking, 15 minutes incline running **STEPPER** **Beginner:** 5 minutes easy pace, 10 minutes high resistance: long, slow steps **Intermediate:** 10 minutes fast pace, 5 minutes high resistance: long, slow steps **Advanced:** 5 minutes fast pace, 10 minutes high resistance: long, slow steps, 5 minutes fast pace
WEDNESDAY	**ROWER** **Beginner:** 5 minutes easy pace, 10 minutes moderate pace **Intermediate:** 10 minutes moderate pace, 5 minutes fast **Advanced:** 3 minutes moderate pace, 2 minutes fast pace: repeat x 3 **STEPPER** **Beginner:** 5 minutes easy pace, 10 minutes high resistance: long, slow steps **Intermediate:** 10 minutes fast pace, 5 minutes high resistance: long, slow steps **Advanced:** 5 minutes fast pace, 10 minutes high resistance: long, slow steps, 5 minutes fast pace
FRIDAY	**SWIMMING** **Beginner:** 20 minutes: 2 lengths fast, 4 lengths recovery **Intermediate:** 30 minutes: 2 lengths fast, 4 lengths recovery, and repeat for duration **Advanced:** 40 minutes: 2 lengths fast, 4 lengths recovery, and repeat for duration
SUNDAY	**RUNNING / WALKING** **Beginner:** 10 minutes incline walking, 5 minutes incline running **Intermediate:** 10 minutes incline walking / running, 10 minutes incline running **Advanced:** 5 minutes incline walking, 15 minutes incline running **ROWER** **Beginner:** 5 minutes easy pace, 10 minutes moderate pace **Intermediate:** 10 minutes moderate pace, 5 minutes fast **Advanced:** 3 minutes moderate pace, 2 minutes fast pace: repeat x 3

WEEK 4

DAY	REPS & ACTIVITY
MONDAY	**STEPPER** **Beginner:** 5 minutes easy pace, 10 minutes high resistance: long, slow steps **Intermediate:** 10 minutes fast pace, 5 minutes high resistance: long, slow steps **Advanced:** 5 minutes fast pace, 10 minutes high resistance: long, slow steps, 5 minutes fast pace **CYCLING** **Beginner:** 5 minutes moderate pace, 5 minutes high resistance, low RPM, 10 minutes moderate pace **Intermediate:** 5 minutes fast pace, 10 minutes high resistance, low RPM, 5 minutes moderate pace **Advanced:** 10 minutes fast pace, 10 minutes high resistance, low RPM, 5 minutes fast pace
WEDNESDAY	**WALKING / RUNNING** **Beginner:** 10 minutes incline walking, 5 minutes incline running **Intermediate:** 10 minutes incline walking / running, 10 minutes incline running **Advanced:** 5 minutes incline walking, 15 minutes incline running **ROWER** **Beginner:** 5 minutes easy pace, 10 minutes moderate pace **Intermediate:** 10 minutes moderate pace, 5 minutes fast pace **Advanced:** 3 minutes moderate pace, 2 minutes fast pace: repeat x 3
FRIDAY	**SWIMMING** **Beginner:** 30 minutes: 2 lengths fast, 4 lengths recovery, and repeat for duration **Intermediate:** 40 minutes: 2 lengths fast, 4 lengths recovery, and repeat for duration **Advanced:** 50 minutes: 2 lengths fast, 4 lengths recovery, and repeat for duration
SUNDAY	**CARDIO MEDLEY** **Beginner:** 10 minutes moderate-resistance cycling, 10 minutes rowing, 10 minutes incline walking **Intermediate:** 10 minutes moderate-resistance cycling, 15 minutes rowing, 15 minutes incline running **Advanced:** 10 minutes moderate-resistance cycling, 15 minutes interval training on rower, 10 minutes fast-incline running, 5 minutes sprint-incline running

33

Apple shapes

IN ADDITION TO THE PROGRAMME BELOW, APPLE SHAPES SHOULD AIM TO COMPLETE THREE BURSTS OF 10 TO 15 MINUTES OF BRISK WALKING EVERY DAY

WEEK 1

DAY	REPS & ACTIVITY
MONDAY	**WALKING / RUNNING** **Beginner:** 20 minutes walking **Intermediate:** 20 minutes walking / running **Advanced:** 20 minutes running **CYCLING** **Beginner:** 15 minutes easy pace **Intermediate:** 15 minutes moderate pace **Advanced:** 10 minutes moderate pace, 5 minutes fast
WEDNESDAY	**WALKING / RUNNING** **Beginner:** 20 minutes walking / running **Intermediate:** 15 minutes walking / running, 5 minutes running **Advanced:** 15 minutes moderate-pace running, 5 minutes fast pace **CYCLING** **Beginner:** 15 minutes easy pace, 5 minutes moderate pace **Intermediate:** 15 minutes moderate pace, 5 minutes fast pace **Advanced:** 10 minutes moderate pace, 10 minutes fast pace
FRIDAY	**WALKING / RUNNING** **Beginner:** 20 minutes walking / running **Intermediate:** 10 minutes walking / running, 10 minutes running **Advanced:** 10 minutes moderate-pace running, 10 minutes fast pace **CYCLING** **Beginner:** 10 minutes easy pace, 10 minutes moderate pace **Intermediate:** 10 minutes moderate pace, 10 minutes fast pace **Advanced:** 5 minutes moderate pace, 15 minutes fast pace
SUNDAY	**WALKING / RUNNING** **Beginner:** 15 minutes walking / running, 5 minutes running **Intermediate:** 5 minutes walking / running, 15 minutes running **Advanced:** 5 minutes moderate-pace running, 5 minutes fast pace, 5 minutes sprinting **CYCLING** **Beginner:** 5 minutes easy pace, 15 minutes moderate pace **Intermediate:** 5 minutes moderate pace, 10 minutes fast pace, 5 minutes moderate pace **Advanced:** 20 minutes fast pace

WEEK 2

DAY	REPS & ACTIVITY
MONDAY	**WALKING / RUNNING** **Beginner:** 15 minutes walking / running, 5 minutes running **Intermediate:** 5 minutes walking / running, 15 minutes running **Advanced:** 5 minutes moderate-pace running, 5 minutes fast pace, 5 minutes sprinting **CROSS-TRAINER** **Beginner:** 15 minutes easy pace **Intermediate:** 15 minutes moderate pace **Advanced:** 10 minutes moderate pace, 5 minutes fast pace
WEDNESDAY	**WALKING / RUNNING** **Beginner:** 15 minutes walking / running, 5 minutes running **Intermediate:** 5 minutes walking / running, 15 minutes running **Advanced:** 5 minutes moderate-pace running, 5 minutes fast pace, 5 minutes sprinting **CROSS-TRAINER** **Beginner:** 15 minutes easy pace, 5 minutes moderate pace **Intermediate:** 15 minutes moderate pace, 5 minutes fast pace **Advanced:** 10 minutes moderate pace, 10 minutes fast pace
FRIDAY	**WALKING / RUNNING** **Beginner:** 15 minutes walking / running, 5 minutes running **Intermediate:** 5 minutes walking / running, 15 minutes running **Advanced:** 5 minutes moderate-pace running, 5 minutes fast pace, 5 minutes sprinting **CROSS-TRAINER** **Beginner:** 10 minutes easy pace, 10 minutes moderate pace **Intermediate:** 10 minutes moderate pace, 10 minutes fast pace **Advanced:** 5 minutes moderate pace, 15 minutes fast pace
SUNDAY	**WALKING / RUNNING** **Beginner:** 10 minutes running **Intermediate:** 20 minutes running **Advanced:** 30 minutes running

WEEK 3

DAY	REPS & ACTIVITY
MONDAY	**CYCLING** **Beginner:** 5 minutes easy pace, 15 minutes moderate pace **Intermediate:** 5 minutes moderate pace, 10 minutes fast pace, 5 minutes moderate pace **Advanced:** 20 minutes fast pace **ROWER** **Beginner:** 15 minutes easy pace **Intermediate:** 10 minutes easy pace, 10 minutes moderate pace **Advanced:** 10 minutes moderate pace, 5 minutes fast pace
WEDNESDAY	**CYCLING** **Beginner:** 5 minutes easy pace, 15 minutes moderate pace **Intermediate:** 5 minutes moderate pace, 10 minutes fast pace, 5 minutes moderate pace **Advanced:** 20 minutes fast pace **ROWER** **Beginner:** 10 minutes easy pace, 5 minutes moderate pace **Intermediate:** 5 minutes easy pace, 15 minutes moderate pace **Advanced:** 10 minutes moderate pace, 10 minutes fast pace
FRIDAY	**CYCLING** **Beginner:** 5 minutes easy pace, 15 minutes moderate pace **Intermediate:** 5 minutes moderate pace, 10 minutes fast pace, 5 minutes moderate pace **Advanced:** 20 minutes fast pace **ROWER** **Beginner:** 10 minutes easy pace, 10 minutes moderate pace **Intermediate:** 20 minutes moderate pace **Advanced:** 5 minutes moderate pace, 5 minutes sprint, 5 minutes moderate pace, 5 minutes sprint
SUNDAY	**CYCLING** **Beginner:** 5 minutes easy pace, 15 minutes moderate pace **Intermediate:** 5 minutes moderate pace, 10 minutes fast pace, 5 minutes moderate pace **Advanced:** 20 minutes fast pace **ROWER** **Beginner:** 5 minutes easy pace, 15 minutes moderate pace **Intermediate:** 15 minutes moderate pace, 5 minutes fast **Advanced:** 5 minutes moderate pace, 10 minutes fast pace, 5 minutes moderate pace, 5 minutes sprint

WEEK 4

DAY	REPS & ACTIVITY
MONDAY	**WALKING / RUNNING** **Beginner:** 10 minutes running **Intermediate:** 20 minutes running **Advanced:** 30 minutes running **CROSS-TRAINER** **Beginner:** 10 minutes easy pace, 10 minutes moderate pace **Intermediate:** 10 minutes moderate pace, 10 minutes fast pace **Advanced:** 5 minutes moderate pace, 15 minutes fast pace
WEDNESDAY	**CYCLING** **Beginner:** 5 minutes easy pace, 15 minutes moderate pace **Intermediate:** 5 minutes moderate pace, 10 minutes fast pace, 5 minutes moderate pace **Advanced:** 20 minutes fast pace **ROWER** **Beginner:** 5 minutes easy pace, 15 minutes moderate pace **Intermediate:** 15 minutes moderate pace, 5 minutes fast pace **Advanced:** 5 minutes moderate pace, 10 minutes fast pace, 5 minutes moderate pace, 5 minutes sprint
FRIDAY	**WALKING / RUNNING** **Beginner:** 15 minutes running **Intermediate:** 25 minutes running **Advanced:** 40 minutes running **CROSS-TRAINER** **Beginner:** 5 minutes easy pace, 15 minutes moderate pace **Intermediate:** 5 minutes moderate pace, 15 minutes fast pace **Advanced:** 20 minutes fast pace
SUNDAY	**CYCLING** **Beginner:** 5 minutes moderate pace, 5 minutes fast pace, 5 minutes moderate pace, 5 minutes fast pace **Intermediate:** 5 minutes moderate pace, 15 minutes fast pace, 5 minutes moderate pace **Advanced:** 25 minutes fast pace **ROWER** **Beginner:** 5 minutes easy pace, 10 minutes moderate pace, 5 minutes fast pace **Intermediate:** 10 minutes moderate pace, 10 minutes fast pace **Advanced:** 5 minutes moderate pace, 15 minutes fast pace, 5 minutes moderate pace

Pear shapes

IN ADDITION TO THE PROGRAMME BELOW, PEAR SHAPES SHOULD AIM TO COMPLETE 30 MINUTES OF BRISK WALKING EVERY DAY

36

WEEK 1

DAY	REPS & ACTIVITY
MONDAY	**WALKING / RUNNING** **Beginner:** 20 minutes walking **Intermediate:** 20 minutes walking / running **Advanced:** 20 minutes running
WEDNESDAY	**CROSS-TRAINER** **Beginner:** 20 minutes easy pace **Intermediate:** 20 minutes moderate pace **Advanced:** 5 minutes moderate pace, 5 minutes fast pace, 5 minutes moderate pace, 5 minutes fast pace **CYCLING** **Beginner:** 20 minutes easy pace **Intermediate:** 20 minutes moderate pace **Advanced:** 5 minutes moderate pace, 5 minutes fast pace, 5 minutes moderate pace, 5 minutes fast pace
FRIDAY	**ROWER** **Beginner:** 15 minutes easy pace **Intermediate:** 10 minutes easy pace, 10 minutes moderate pace **Advanced:** 10 minutes moderate pace, 5 minutes fast pace **WALKING / RUNNING** **Beginner:** 20 minutes walking **Intermediate:** 30 minutes jogging **Advanced:** 20 minutes running
SUNDAY	**SWIMMING** **Beginner:** 30 minutes steady swimming **Intermediate:** 40 minutes steady swimming **Advanced:** 50 minutes steady swimming

WEEK 2

DAY	REPS & ACTIVITY
MONDAY	**WALKING / RUNNING** **Beginner:** 10 minutes walking, 10 minutes walking / running **Intermediate:** 25 minutes walking / running **Advanced:** 20 minutes running – 4 minutes steady speed, 1 minute fast: repeat x 4
WEDNESDAY	**CROSS-TRAINER** **Beginner:** 25 minutes easy pace **Intermediate:** 25 minutes moderate pace **Advanced:** 5 minutes moderate pace, 5 minutes fast pace, 5 minutes moderate pace, 10 minutes fast pace **RUNNING** **Beginner:** 25 minutes easy pace **Intermediate:** 25 minutes moderate pace **Advanced:** 5 minutes moderate pace, 5 minutes fast pace, 5 minutes moderate pace, 10 minutes fast pace
FRIDAY	**ROWER** **Beginner:** 10 minutes easy pace, 5 minutes moderate pace **Intermediate:** 5 minutes easy pace, 15 minutes moderate pace **Advanced:** 10 minutes moderate pace, 10 minutes fast pace **WALKING / RUNNING** **Beginner:** 10 minutes walking, 10 minutes walking / running **Intermediate:** 25 minutes walking / running **Advanced:** 20 minutes running – 4 minutes steady speed, 1 minute fast: repeat x 4
SUNDAY	**SWIMMING** **Beginner:** 30 minutes steady swimming with 1 fast length every 4 **Intermediate:** 40 minutes steady swimming with 1 fast length every 4 **Advanced:** 50 minutes steady swimming with 1 fast length every 4

WEEK 3

DAY	REPS & ACTIVITY
MONDAY	**WALKING / RUNNING** **Beginner:** 10 minutes walking, 15 minutes walking / running **Intermediate:** 30 minutes walking / running **Advanced:** 30 minutes running – 4 minutes steady speed, 1 minute fast: repeat x 6
WEDNESDAY	**CROSS-TRAINER** **Beginner:** 15 minutes easy pace, 5 minutes moderate pace **Intermediate:** 20 minutes moderate pace, 5 minutes fast **Advanced:** 5 minutes moderate pace, 10 minutes fast pace, 5 minutes moderate pace, 10 minutes fast pace **CYCLING** **Beginner:** 15 minutes easy pace, 5 minutes moderate pace **Intermediate:** 20 minutes moderate pace, 5 minutes fast pace **Advanced:** 5 minutes moderate pace, 10 minutes fast pace, 5 minutes moderate pace, 10 minutes fast pace
FRIDAY	**ROWER** **Beginner:** 10 minutes easy pace, 10 minutes moderate pace **Intermediate:** 20 minutes moderate pace **Advanced:** 5 minutes moderate pace, 5 minutes sprint, 5 minutes moderate pace, 5 minutes sprint **WALKING / RUNNING** **Beginner:** 10 minutes walking, 15 minutes walking / running **Intermediate:** 30 minutes walking / running **Advanced:** 30 minutes running – 4 minutes steady speed, 1 minute fast: repeat x 6
SUNDAY	**SWIMMING** **Beginner:** 30 minutes steady swimming with 2 fast lengths every 6 **Intermediate:** 40 minutes steady swimming with 2 fast lengths every 6 **Advanced:** 50 minutes steady swimming with 2 fast lengths every 6

WEEK 4

DAY	REPS & ACTIVITY
MONDAY	**WALKING / RUNNING** **Beginner:** 10 minutes walking, 20 minutes walking / running **Intermediate:** 20 minutes walking, 10 minutes running **Advanced:** 30 minutes running – 3 minutes steady speed, 2 minutes fast: repeat x 6
WEDNESDAY	**CROSS-TRAINER** **Beginner:** 10 minutes easy pace, 10 minutes moderate pace **Intermediate:** 15 minutes moderate pace, 10 minutes fast pace **Advanced:** 30 minutes – 5 minutes moderate pace, 20 minutes fast pace, 5 minutes moderate pace **CYCLING** **Beginner:** 10 minutes easy pace, 10 minutes moderate pace **Intermediate:** 15 minutes moderate pace, 10 minutes fast pace **Advanced:** 5 minutes moderate pace, 20 minutes fast pace, 5 minutes moderate pace
FRIDAY	**ROWER** **Beginner:** 5 minutes easy pace, 5 minutes moderate pace **Intermediate:** 15 minutes moderate pace, 5 minutes fast pace **Advanced:** 5 minutes moderate pace, 10 minutes fast pace, 5 minutes moderate pace, 5 minutes sprint **WALKING / RUNNING** **Beginner:** 10 minutes walking, 20 minutes walking / running **Intermediate:** 20 minutes walking, 10 minutes running **Advanced:** 30 minutes running – 3 minutes steady speed, 2 minutes fast: repeat x 6
SUNDAY	**SWIMMING** **Beginner:** 40 minutes steady swimming **Intermediate:** 50 minutes steady swimming **Advanced:** 60 minutes steady swimming

The importance of stretching

DON'T FORGET THAT WARMING UP BEFORE YOU EXERCISE AND COOLING DOWN AFTERWARDS IS VITAL EVERY TIME YOU WORK OUT

38

Muscles warm up like chewing gum, and if you exercise while they are still cold and stiff, they will be more susceptible to injury. However, if you warm them up before you work out, by doing a milder form of the exercise you are about to do – for example, jogging for five minutes before you go on a 20-minute run – then they will respond better for the rest of the session.

Dynamic stretching (stretching with movement) is also useful pre-exercise, as it raises the heart rate, which in turn increases the blood flow to the muscles and the synovial fluid around the joints, widens your range of movement and prepares you mentally for the exercise you are about to perform. Dynamic stretches include hamstring curls, squats and heel digs.

Equally, after you have worked out, it is important to stretch the muscles back to their pre-exercise length. This type of stretching is known as developmental, and it improves flexibility and increases muscle length. Larger muscles, for example, the hamstrings (back of the legs) and quads (front of the thighs), will need to be stretched for 15 to 30 seconds. Initially, hold the stretch for eight to ten seconds, and then deepen the stretch when you feel the tension in the muscle ease. Remember to always breathe out as you stretch.

And don't forget – never force a stretch or continue one if it is painful.

> 'If you warm up your muscles before you work out (by doing a milder form of the exercise you are about to do) then they respond better to exercise'

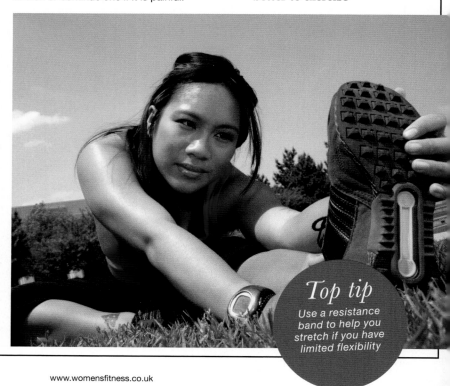

Top tip
Use a resistance band to help you stretch if you have limited flexibility

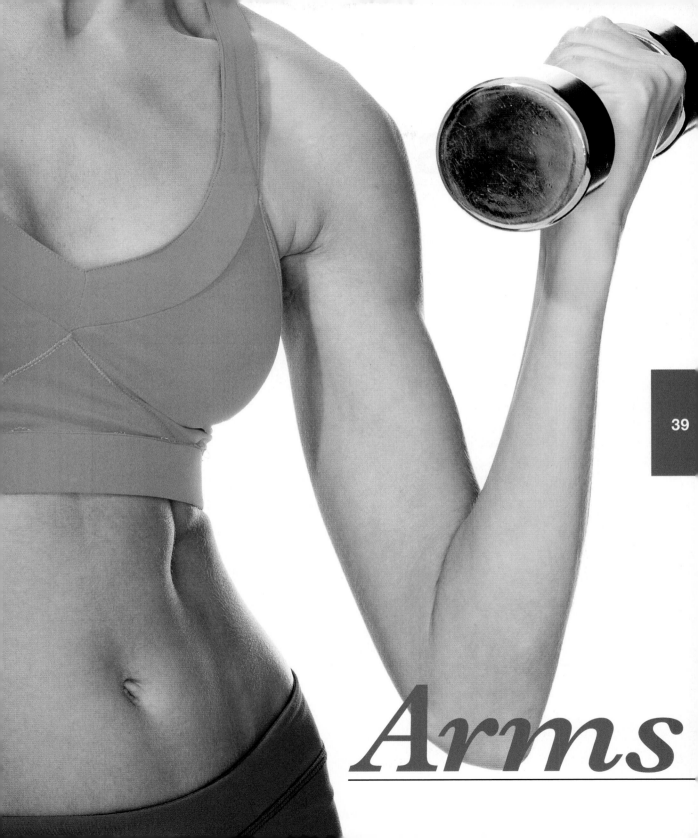

Arms

ARMS GUIDELINES

About the arms
Toned arms are a great asset if you want to wear sleeveless tops and dresses. Apple and hourglass bodyshapes usually have to work harder to achieve them, so it's important for these shapes to include two exercises for the back and front of the arms in each workout to maximise results.

Use a 2kg pair of dumbbells for all exercises that include weights

APPLE

	REPS
BEGINNER	2 sets of 15 reps
INTERMEDIATE	2 sets of 20 reps
ADVANCED	3 sets of 20 reps

PEAR

	REPS
BEGINNER	2 sets of 10 reps
INTERMEDIATE	2 sets of 15 reps
ADVANCED	2 sets of 20 reps

HOURGLASS

	REPS
BEGINNER	2 sets of 15 reps
INTERMEDIATE	2 sets of 20 reps
ADVANCED	3 sets of 20 reps

BOY

	REPS
BEGINNER	2 sets of 10 reps
INTERMEDIATE	2 sets of 15 reps
ADVANCED	2 sets of 20 reps

BICEPS CURL

Apple, hourglass, boy, pear

Area trained: Biceps
Technique:
★ Stand with your feet hip-width apart, holding a weight in each hand.
★ Keep a slight bend in your elbows, and your palms facing forward. This is the start position.
★ Keeping your elbows tucked into your sides, curl your arms up to your shoulders.
★ Slowly lower your arms back to the start position and repeat.

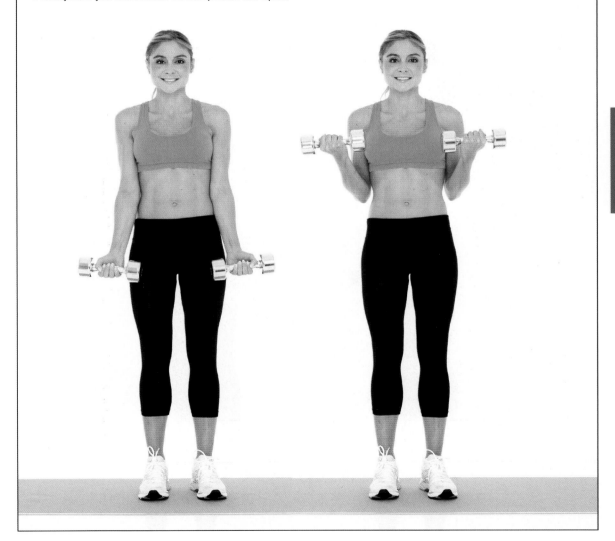

41

ALTERNATING HAMMER CURL

Apple, hourglass, boy, pear

Area trained: Biceps
Technique:
★ Stand with your feet hip-width apart, holding a weight in each hand.
★ Keep a slight bend in your elbows, with your palms facing in and your thumbs forward. This is the start position.
★ Keeping your elbows tucked into your sides, slowly curl your right arm up to your shoulder.
★ Slowly lower the weight back to the start position and repeat with the left arm.
★ Alternate between right and left. One on each arm is one repetition.

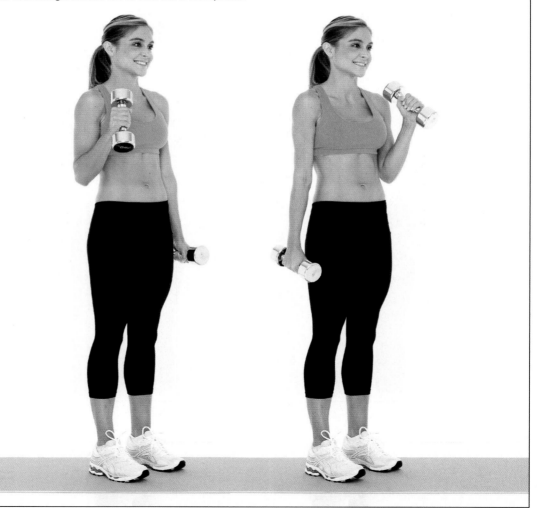

42

REVERSE CURL

Apple, hourglass, boy, pear

Area trained: Biceps
Technique:
★ Stand with your feet hip-width apart, holding a weight in each hand, with your palms facing the floor. This is the start position.
★ Keeping your elbows tucked into your sides, curl your arms up to your shoulders with your palms facing away from you.
★ Slowly lower your arms back to the start position and repeat.

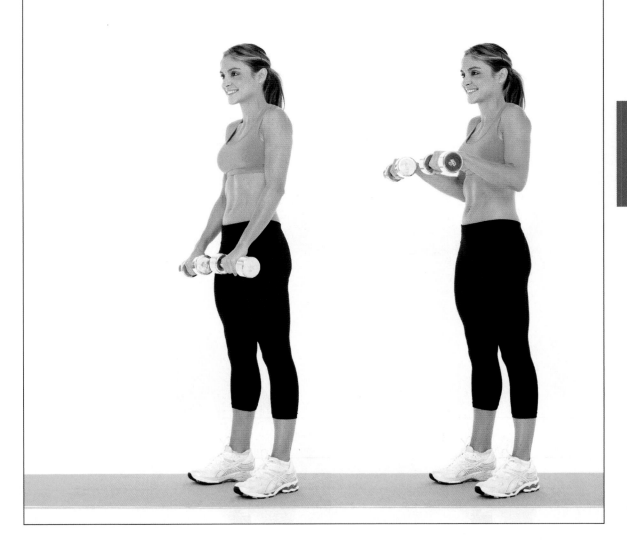

43

LYING TRICEPS EXTENSION

Apple, hourglass, boy, pear

Area trained: Triceps
Technique:
★ Lie on your back, holding a weight in each hand.
★ Stretch out your arms so the weights are on the floor above your head, and your palms are facing each other. This is the start position.
★ Extend your arms upwards but don't lock your elbows.
★ Ensure that you keep your shoulders still throughout the movement.
★ Lower the weights back to the start position, but don't rest them on the floor and repeat.

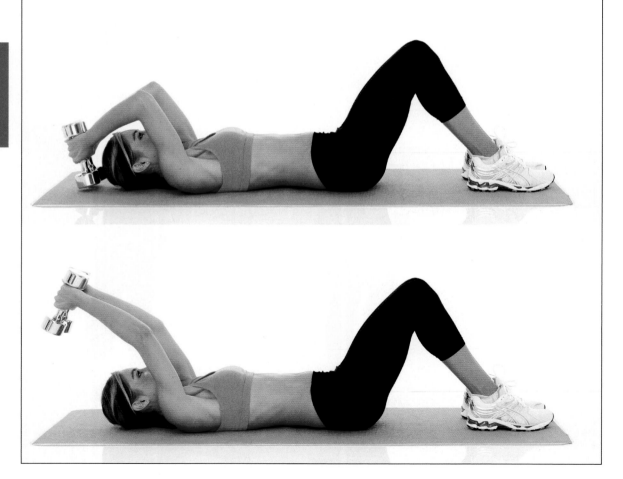

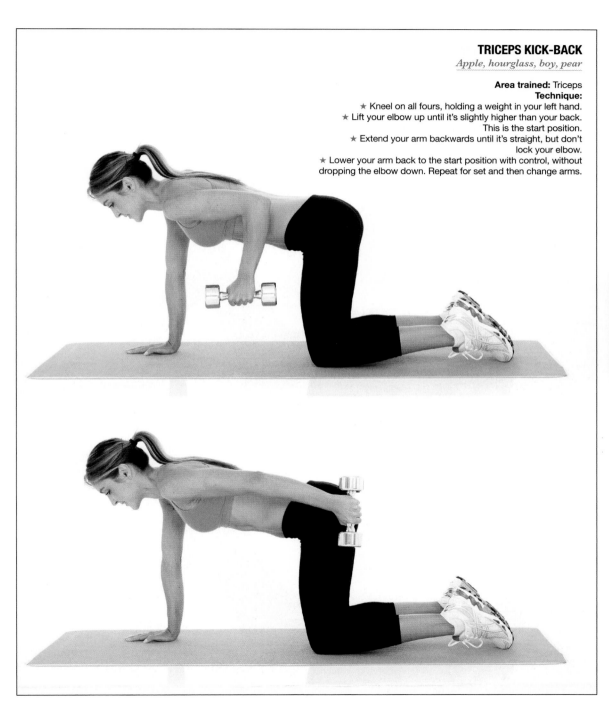

TRICEPS KICK-BACK
Apple, hourglass, boy, pear

Area trained: Triceps
Technique:
★ Kneel on all fours, holding a weight in your left hand.
★ Lift your elbow up until it's slightly higher than your back. This is the start position.
★ Extend your arm backwards until it's straight, but don't lock your elbow.
★ Lower your arm back to the start position with control, without dropping the elbow down. Repeat for set and then change arms.

45

SINGLE DUMBBELL CHEST PRESS

Apple, hourglass, boy, pear

Areas trained: Triceps and chest
Technique:
★ Lie on your back, holding one dumbbell with both hands.
★ Keep your elbows by your sides. This is the start position.
★ Extend your arms up to the ceiling, but don't lock your elbows.
★ Lower your arms back to the start position, until your elbows touch the floor and repeat.

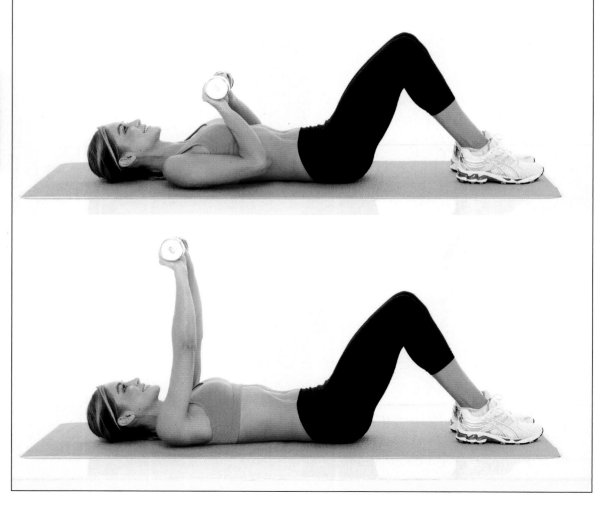

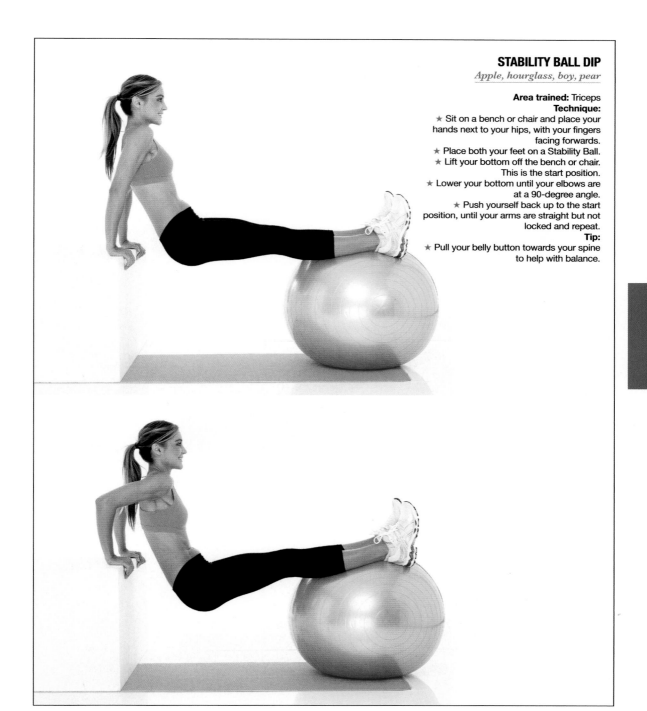

STABILITY BALL DIP

Apple, hourglass, boy, pear

Area trained: Triceps

Technique:

★ Sit on a bench or chair and place your hands next to your hips, with your fingers facing forwards.

★ Place both your feet on a Stability Ball.

★ Lift your bottom off the bench or chair. This is the start position.

★ Lower your bottom until your elbows are at a 90-degree angle.

★ Push yourself back up to the start position, until your arms are straight but not locked and repeat.

Tip:

★ Pull your belly button towards your spine to help with balance.

47

DIAMOND PRESS-UP

Apple, hourglass, boy, pear

Areas trained: Triceps, chest and shoulders
Technique:
★ Kneel on all fours.
★ Place your hands close together to form a diamond with your index fingers and thumbs (as pictured).
★ Bend your elbows and lower your upper body to the floor.
★ Push up and extend your arms. Repeat.

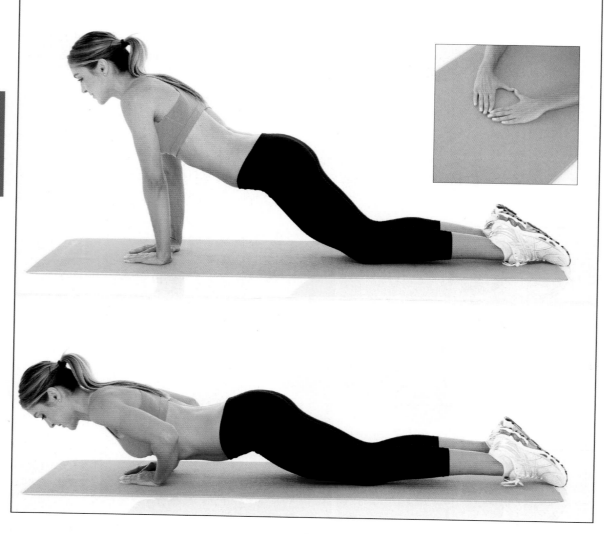

48

ELASTIC BAND TRICEPS PRESS-DOWN

Apple, hourglass, boy, pear

Area trained: Triceps
Technique:
★ Hold an elasticated band in your left hand and extend your left arm up to the ceiling.
★ Grab hold of the elasticated band with your right hand.
★ Keep your right elbow bent and tucked into your side. This is the start position.
★ Pull the elastic band down by extending your right arm down towards the floor.
★ Slowly return to the start position.
★ Complete one set before changing over to the other side.

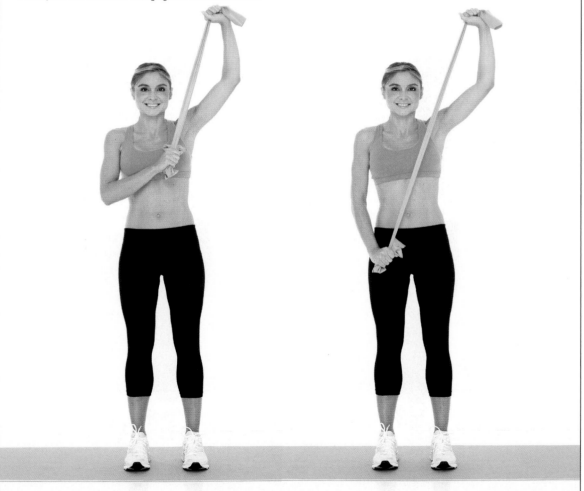

49

ELASTIC BAND OVERHEAD EXTENSION

Apple, hourglass, boy, pear

Area trained: Triceps
Technique:
★ Hold an elasticated band in your right hand and extend your right arm up to the ceiling.
★ Bend your right elbow.
★ Use your left hand to grab hold of the band behind your back.
★ Extend your right arm up while keeping your elbow next to your ear.
★ Lower with control.
★ Complete one set before changing over to the other side.

50

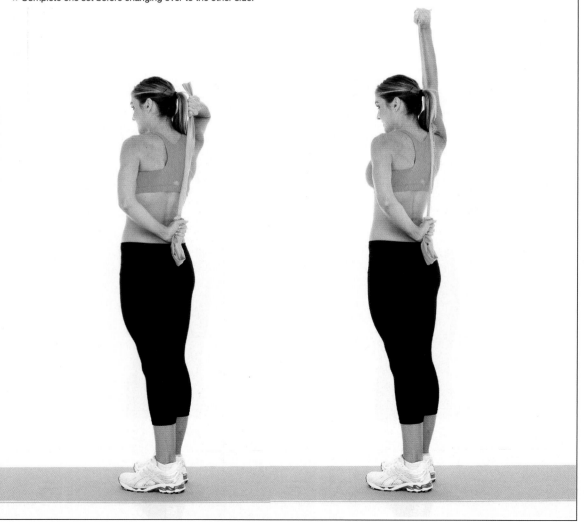

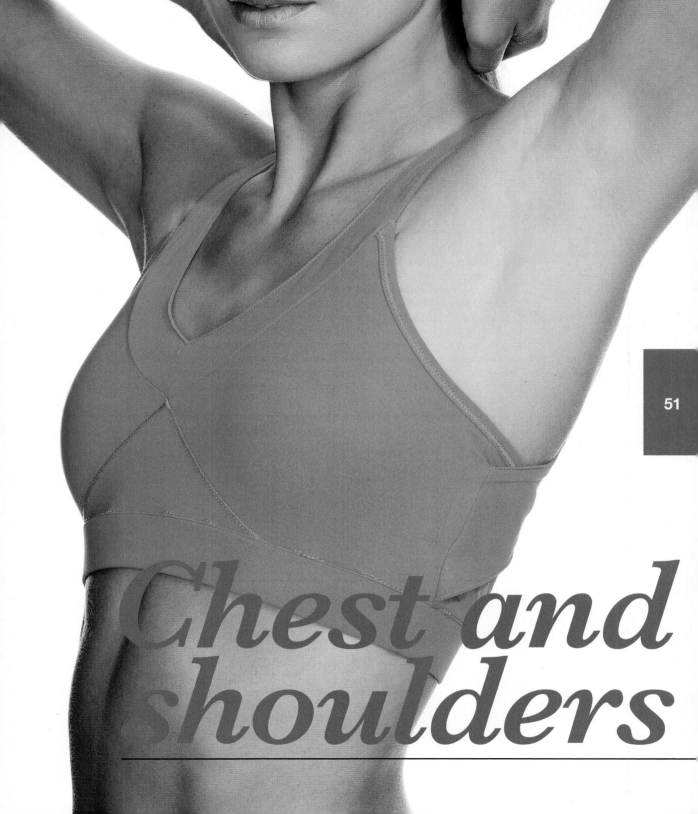

Chest and shoulders

CHEST AND SHOULDERS GUIDELINES

About the chest and shoulders

Chest exercises can really help to improve the appearance of your bust and reduce the risk of developing sagging breasts, so if you want to firm up this area, it's very important to include them in your workout. Toning up your shoulders, especially the back area, will improve your posture and reduce the flabby bit around your armpits, and having toned chest and shoulder muscles will boost your confidence when wearing your favourite strapless dress. Women with hourglass and boy shapes should include more than one exercise from this section in their workout: if you have a boy bodyshape and are prone to picking up muscle weight quickly, keep the weights low, even if it feels quite easy.

Use a 2kg pair of dumbbells for all exercises that include weights

52

APPLE

	REPS
BEGINNER	2 sets of 10 reps
INTERMEDIATE	2 sets of 15 reps
ADVANCED	2 sets of 20 reps

PEAR

	REPS
BEGINNER	2 sets of 10 reps
INTERMEDIATE	2 sets of 15 reps
ADVANCED	2 sets of 20 reps

HOURGLASS

	REPS
BEGINNER	2 sets of 15 reps
INTERMEDIATE	2 sets of 20 reps
ADVANCED	3 sets of 20 reps

BOY

	REPS
BEGINNER	2 sets of 15 reps
INTERMEDIATE	2 sets of 20 reps
ADVANCED	3 sets of 20 reps

V-FLY

Hourglass, boy, apple, pear

Areas trained: Chest and arms
Technique:
★ Lie on your back holding a weight in each hand.
★ Extend your arms up to the ceiling.
★ Form a V-position with the weights. This is the start position.
★ Lower the weights to the floor. Lift the weights back up to the start position and repeat.
Tips:
★ Keep the weights over your chest and not your face.
★ Always keep a slight bend in your elbows.

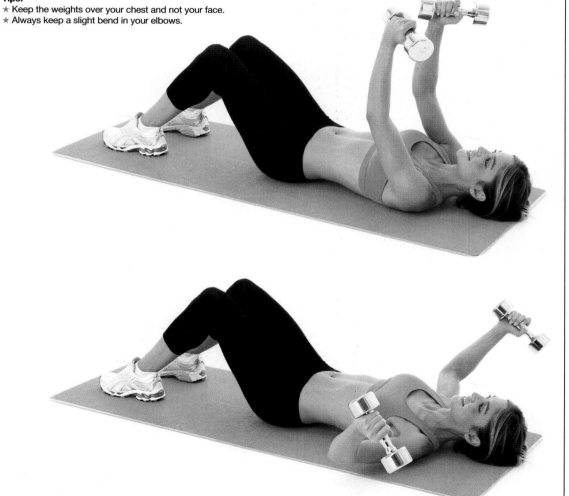

STABILITY BALL PRESS-UP WITH HANDS ON FLOOR

Hourglass, boy, apple, pear

Areas trained: Chest, arms and core
Technique:
★ Place your hands on the floor and your legs on a Stability Ball.
★ Keep your hands slightly wider than shoulder-width. This is the start position.
★ Bend your elbows and lower your chest to the floor.
★ Keep your back straight and your tummy tight.
★ Straighten your arms and return to the start position. Repeat.
Tip:
★ If your back hurts you are arching your back, so lift your bottom higher.

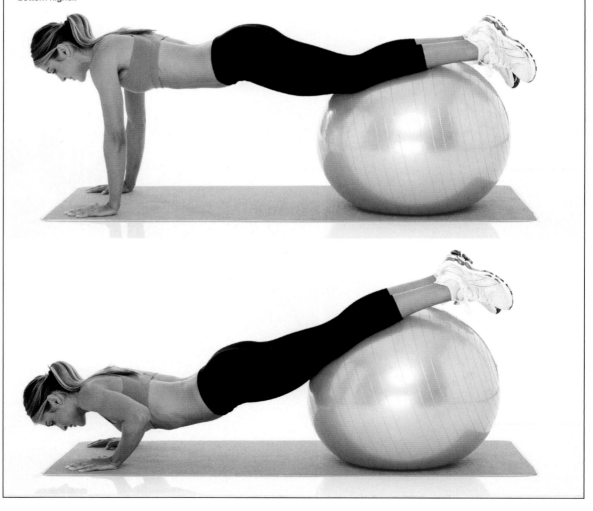

54

STABILITY BALL PRESS-UP WITH HANDS ON BALL (ADVANCED)

Hourglass, boy, apple, pear

Areas trained: Chest, arms and core
Technique:
★ Lie with your chest on a Stability Ball.
★ Place your hands next to your shoulders on the Stability Ball, keeping your fingers spread open. This is the start position.
★ Keep your legs wide to aid balance.
★ Straighten your arms and lift your body off the ball.
★ Lower back to the start position with control. Repeat.

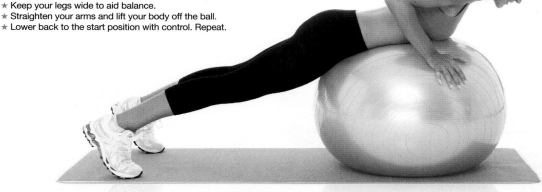

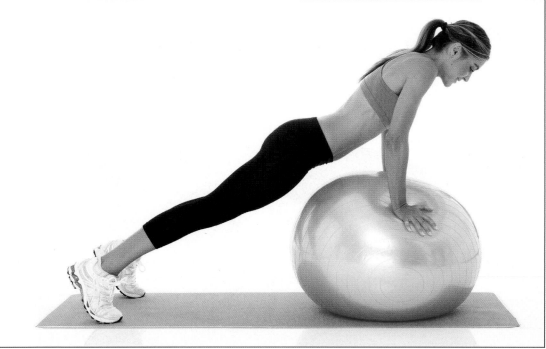

55

STABILITY BALL PULLOVER
Hourglass, boy, apple, pear

Area trained: Chest
Technique:
★ Lie with your head and shoulders on a Stability Ball, holding a weight in each hand.
★ Extend your arms up to the ceiling, with a slight bend in your elbows and your palms facing away from you. This is the start position.
★ Lower your arms over your head until your arms are next to your ears.
★ Lift up and return to the start position. Repeat.

Tip:
★ Only lower as far as your shoulder flexibility will allow you.
★ Keep the same angle in your elbows throughout the movement.

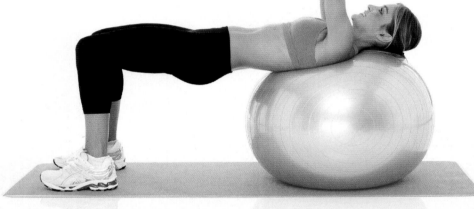

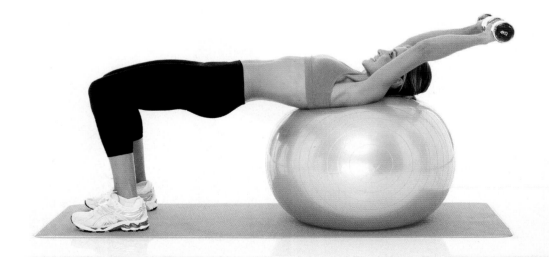

DUMBBELL CHEST PRESS

Hourglass, boy, apple, pear

Areas trained: Chest and arms
Technique:
★ Lie on your back holding a weight in each hand, with your palms facing towards your feet.
★ Extend your arms up to the ceiling.
★ Lower the weights until your elbows touch the floor.
★ Lift up and return to the start position and repeat.

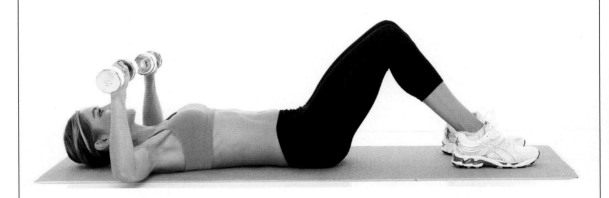

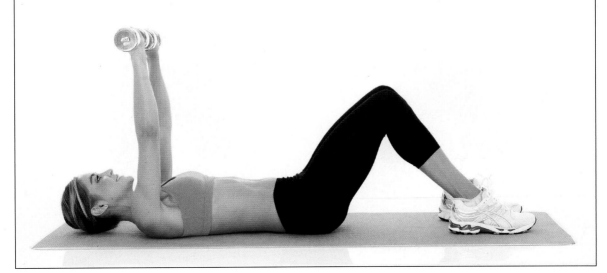

SEATED SHOULDER PRESS
Hourglass, boy, apple, pear

Area trained: Shoulders
Technique:
★ Sit on a Stability Ball with your feet shoulder-width apart.
★ Hold a weight in each hand at the same level as your shoulders, with your palms facing forward.
★ Extend your arms up without locking them.
★ Lower with control until the weights are back level with your shoulders again. Repeat.

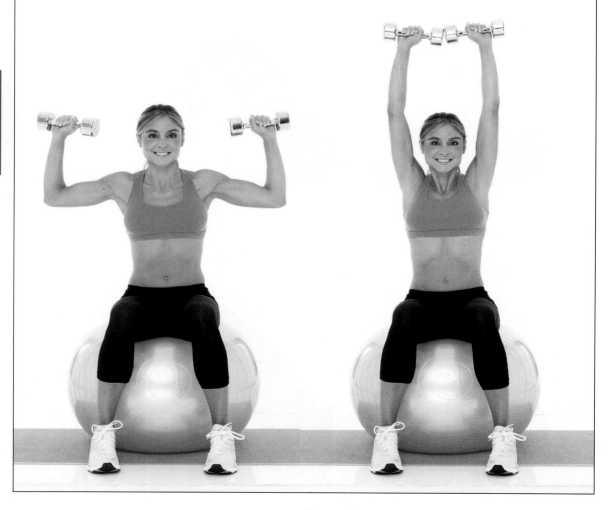

DUMBBELL SIDE RAISES
Hourglass, boy, apple, pear

Area trained: Shoulders
Technique:
★ Stand with feet slightly wider than hip-width apart.
★ Holding a weight in each hand, bend your elbows 90 degrees, with your palms facing each other.
★ Lift your arms sideways until your hands, elbows and shoulders are level. Lower with control and repeat.

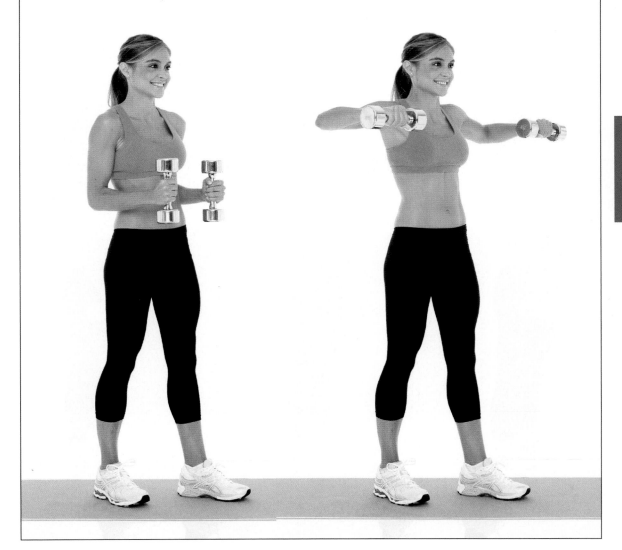

59

SINGLE ARM FRONT RAISES

Hourglass, boy, apple, pear

Area trained: Shoulders
Technique:
★ Stand with your feet hip-width apart, holding a weight in each hand, with your palms facing down.
★ Keep your arms in front of your thighs and a slight bend in your elbows.
★ Lift your left arm up to shoulder height.
★ Lower with control and repeat with your right arm. This is one rep.
Tip:
★ Ensure that you don't swing your body to lift the weight up.

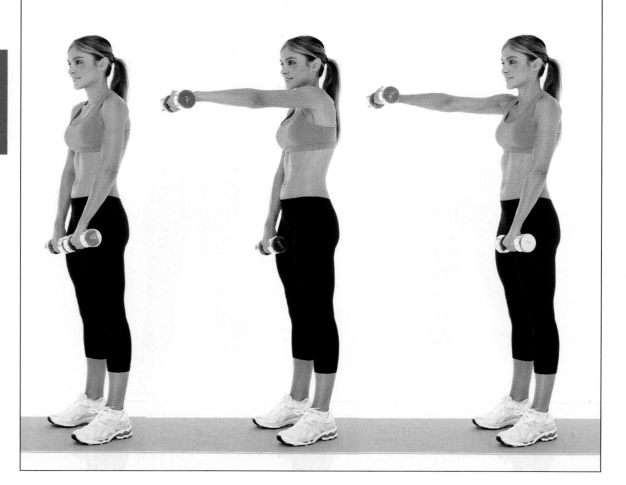

BEND-OVER FLY

Hourglass, boy, apple, pear

Area trained: Shoulders
Technique:
★ Stand with your right leg in front of your left leg.
★ Hold a weight in each hand, with your palms facing each other.
★ Keep a slight bend in your arms.
★ Lift your arms sideways until your hands are level with your shoulders.
★ Lower with control. Repeat.

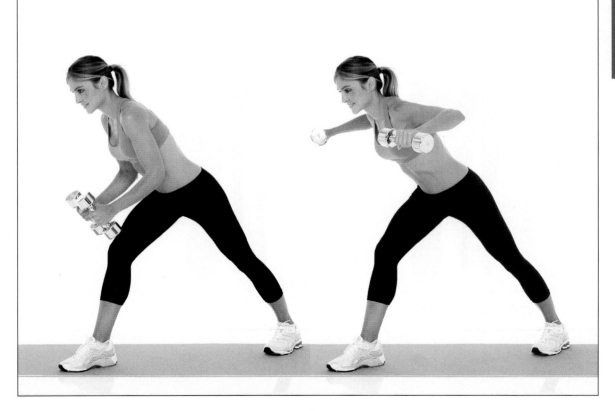

ELASTIC BAND DIAGONAL RAISE

Hourglass, boy, apple, pear

Area trained: Shoulders
Technique:
★ Stand upright with your feet shoulder-width apart.
★ Hold the end of an elasticated band in your left hand, keeping your right arm by your side.
★ Grab hold of the middle of the elasticated band with your right hand, keeping it facing down towards your legs. This is the start position.
★ Maintaining a slight bend in your right elbow, lift your left arm diagonally up to shoulder level.
★ Slowly return to the start position. Complete one set before repeating on the other side.

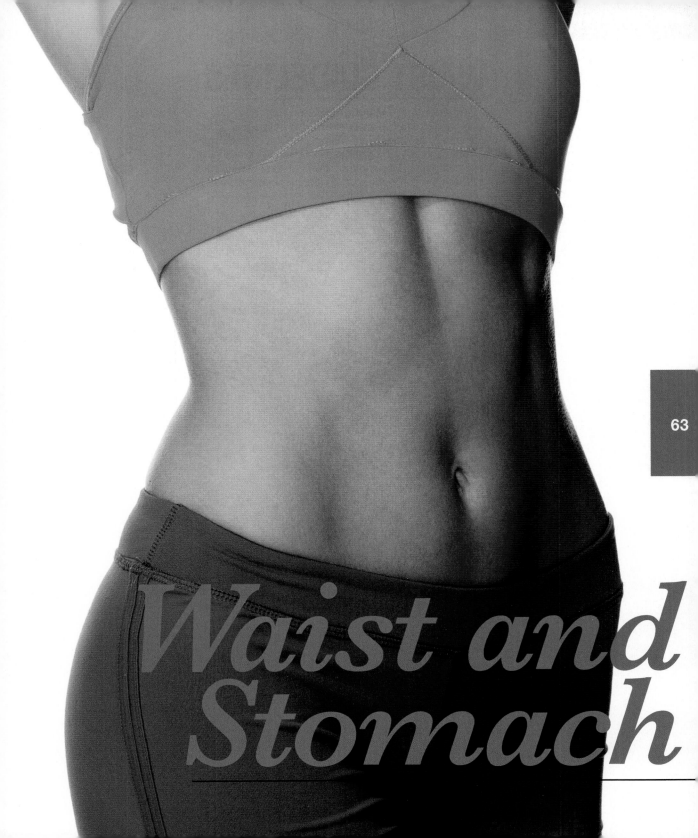

Waist and Stomach

WAIST GUIDELINES

About the waist

Doing waist exercises will help you to shape and tone your waistline. Waist exercises are particularly important for apple and boy bodyshapes, so if you fall into either of these categories, you should include at least two to three of these in each workout, with a high number of reps.

APPLE

	REPS
BEGINNER	2 sets of 15 reps
INTERMEDIATE	2 sets of 20 reps
ADVANCED	2 sets of 30 reps

PEAR

	REPS
BEGINNER	2 sets of 10 reps
INTERMEDIATE	2 sets of 15 reps
ADVANCED	2 sets of 20 reps

HOURGLASS

	REPS
BEGINNER	2 sets of 10 reps
INTERMEDIATE	2 sets of 15 reps
ADVANCED	2 sets of 20 reps

BOY

	REPS
BEGINNER	2 sets of 15 reps
INTERMEDIATE	2 sets of 20 reps
ADVANCED	2 sets of 30 reps

64

STOMACH GUIDELINES

About the stomach

Stomach exercises can make a big difference to most bodies, especially as we get older. Women with apple and boy bodyshapes will have to work harder for a flat stomach than those with hourglass and pear shapes, so apples and boys should include at least two to three of these stomach exercises in their workout.

APPLE

	REPS
BEGINNER	2 sets of 15 reps
INTERMEDIATE	2 sets of 20 reps
ADVANCED	2 sets of 30 reps

PEAR

	REPS
BEGINNER	2 sets of 10 reps
INTERMEDIATE	2 sets of 15 reps
ADVANCED	2 sets of 20 reps

HOURGLASS

	REPS
BEGINNER	2 sets of 10 reps
INTERMEDIATE	2 sets of 15 reps
ADVANCED	2 sets of 20 reps

BOY

	REPS
BEGINNER	2 sets of 15 reps
INTERMEDIATE	2 sets of 20 reps
ADVANCED	2 sets of 30 reps

SIDE-ISOLATED CRUNCH

Apple, boy, pear and hourglass

Areas trained: Stomach and side muscles
Technique:
★ Lie down on your back with your knees bent.
★ Place your left hand behind your head and extend your right arm out straight, next to your body.
★ Lift your shoulders and left arm off the floor.
★ Crunch sideways, reaching your right hand towards your right foot.
★ Return to the centre position and lower your shoulders back to the floor.
★ Complete one set on the left side and then repeat on the right side.

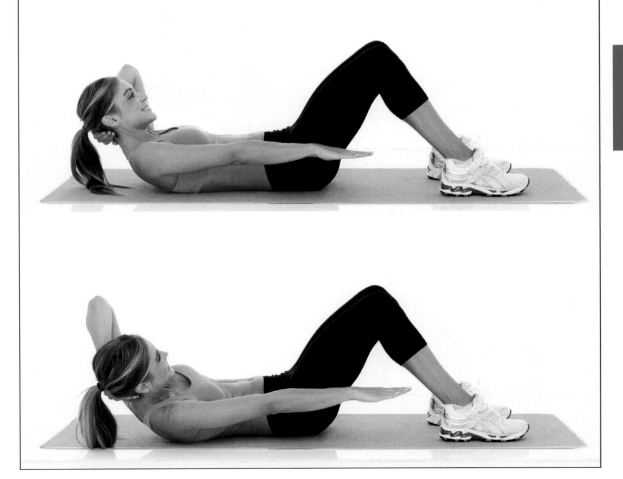

SIDE CRUNCH

Apple, boy, pear and hourglass

Area trained: Waist
Technique:
★ Lie on your side with your hands behind your head.
★ Lift your feet off the floor.
★ Tuck your knees in until they touch your top elbow.
★ Extend your legs again.
★ Complete one set before repeating on the other side.

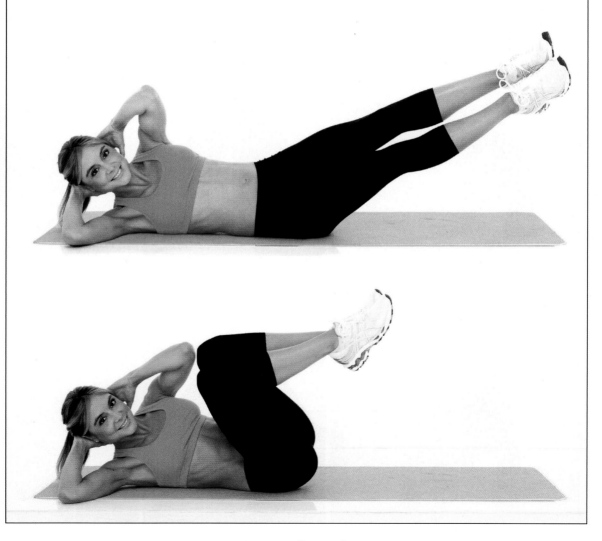

SIDE PLANK LIFT

Apple, boy, pear and hourglass

Area trained: Side muscles
Technique:
★ Lie on your right side with your left foot on top of your right.
★ Place your right elbow directly underneath your right shoulder.
★ Lift your hips off the floor until you have a straight line between your shoulders, hips and feet.
★ Lower your hips to touch the floor, but don't rest them on the floor.
★ Complete one set on the right side before changing over to the left side.

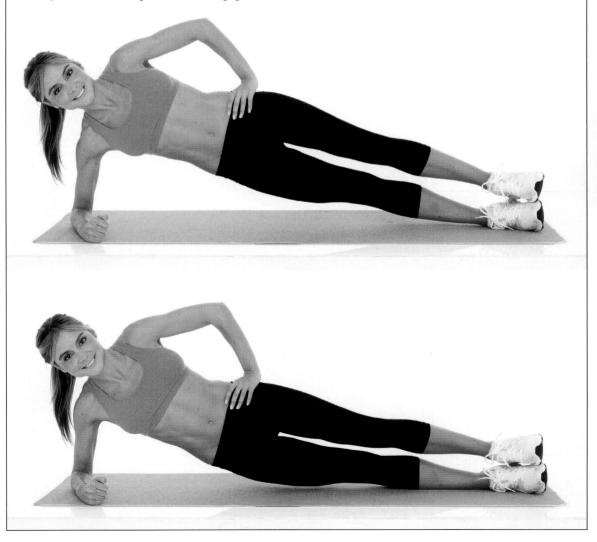

THREADING NEEDLE

Apple, boy, pear and hourglass

Areas trained: Side muscles, core and balance
Technique:
★ Lie in a straight line on your left side.
★ Place your left elbow directly underneath your left shoulder and extend your right arm up to the ceiling.
★ Lift your hips off the floor into the side plank position. This is the start position.
★ Lower your right arm and thread it between your left arm and the floor.
★ Complete one set before repeating on the other side.

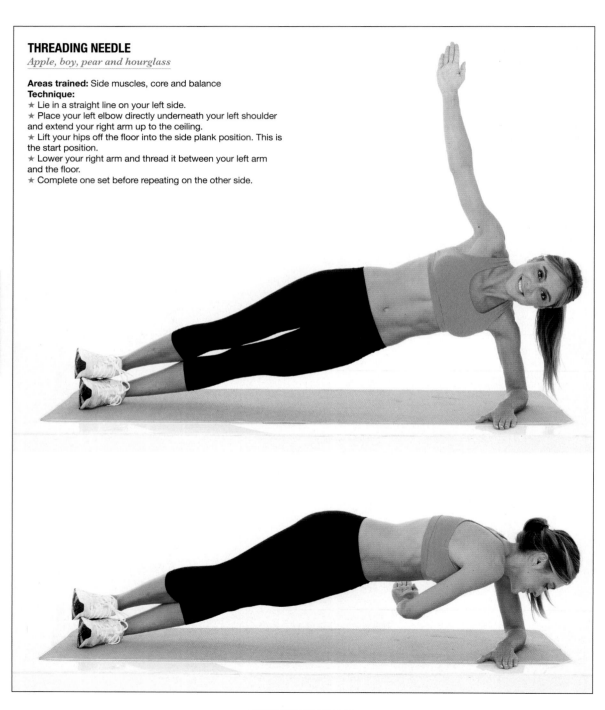

MEDICINE BALL SIDE LEG LIFT

Apple, boy, pear and hourglass

Areas trained: Side muscles and inner thighs
Technique:
★ Lie on your side and place a Medicine ball in between your knees.
★ Place your top hand on the floor for balance.
★ Lift your legs off the floor, keeping them straight.
★ Lower with control. Complete one set and repeat on the other side.

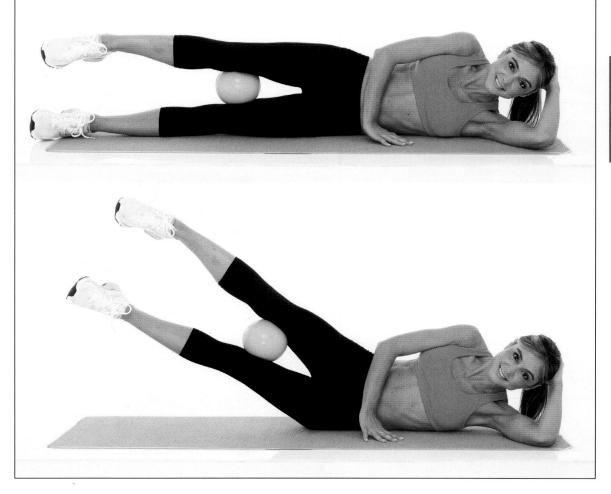

SEATED MEDICINE BALL ROTATION
Apple, boy, pear and hourglass

Area trained: Side muscles
Technique:
★ Sit on the floor with your legs wide apart.
★ Hold a Medicine ball (or any appropriate weight) in front of your chest.
★ Rotate your upper body towards the left.
★ Rotate your upper body towards the right.
★ Repeat, alternating between left and right.
Note:
★ Doing this exercise in the seated position helps to keep your hips still throughout the range of motion.

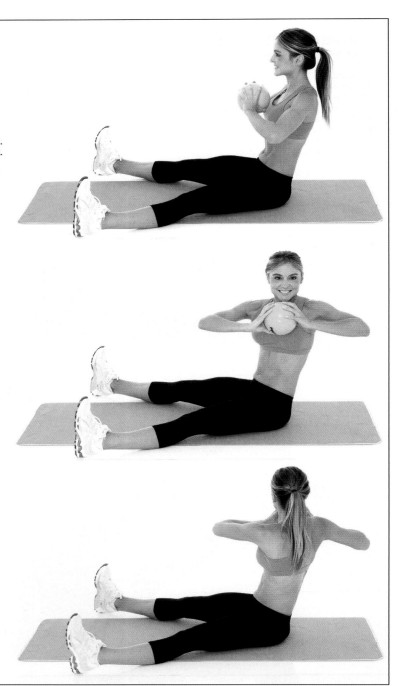

V-SIT MEDICINE BALL ROTATION

Apple, boy, pear, hourglass

Areas trained: Side muscles and core
Technique:
★ Sit on the floor with your knees bent, holding a Medicine ball in front of your chest.
★ Lift both feet off the floor.
★ Lower your upper body backwards until you feel tension in your stomach.
★ Hold this position while rotating the Medicine ball towards your left side.
★ Let the ball touch the floor but don't rest it there.
★ Rotate over to the right side.
★ Repeat, alternating between left and right.
Tip:
★ Don't hold your breath.

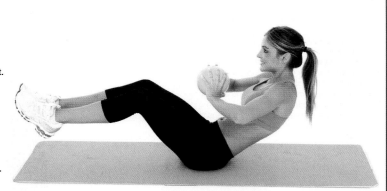

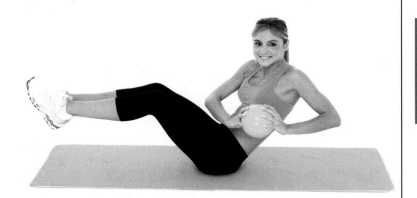

71

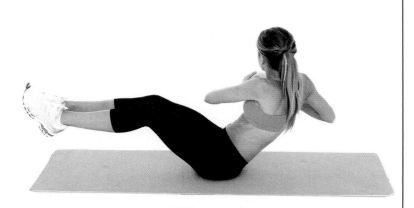

STRAIGHT-LEG HIP-ROLL

Apple, boy, pear and hourglass

Area trained: Side muscles
Technique:

★ Lie on your back and extend your legs up to the ceiling, with your arms out to the sides. This is the start position.
★ Roll your legs over to the right until your feet touch the floor.
★ Use your side muscles to lift your legs back up to the start position.
★ Roll over to the left.
★ Repeat, alternating between right and left.

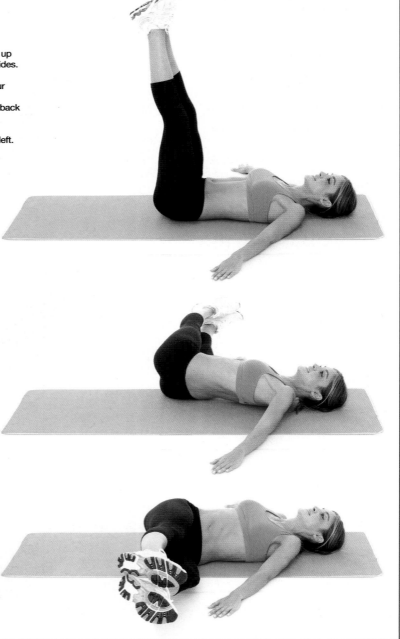

72

FLOOR SIDE-LIFT

Apple, boy, pear and hourglass

Area trained: Side muscles
Technique:
★ Lie on your right side and place your feet against a wall.
★ Keep your knees slightly bent and cross your arms over your chest.
★ Push your legs firmly against the wall while lifting your shoulders off the floor.
★ Lower with control.
★ Repeat one set on the right before changing over to the left.

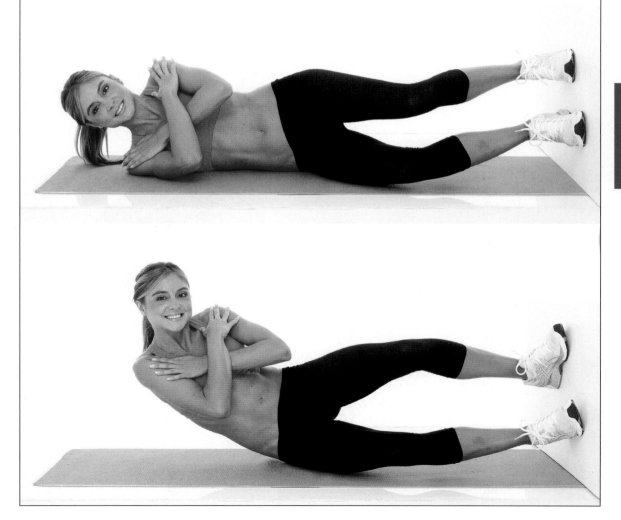

73

SIDE LIFT OVER STABILITY BALL
Apple, boy, pear and hourglass

Area trained: Side muscles
Technique:
★ Sit with your right hip on a Stability Ball.
★ Keeping both feet braced against a wall to help you with your balance, extend your right leg forwards and your left leg backwards.
★ Cross your hands over your chest or hold onto a weight. This is the start position.
★ Lower your body sideways over the ball.
★ Raise yourself back to the start position and repeat, before switching sides.

74

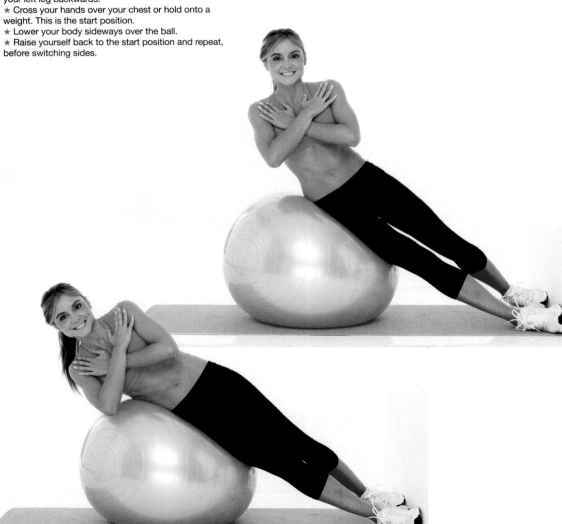

TOE TAP

Apple, boy, pear, hourglass

Area trained: Lower stomach
Technique:
★ Lie on your back with your feet in the air with a
90-degree bend in your knees. This is the start position.
★ Pull your belly button towards your spine.
★ Lower your feet until your toes just touch the floor.
★ Keep your back in a neutral position throughout the range of motion
(don't let it arch upwards).
★ Lift both legs back to the start position and repeat.

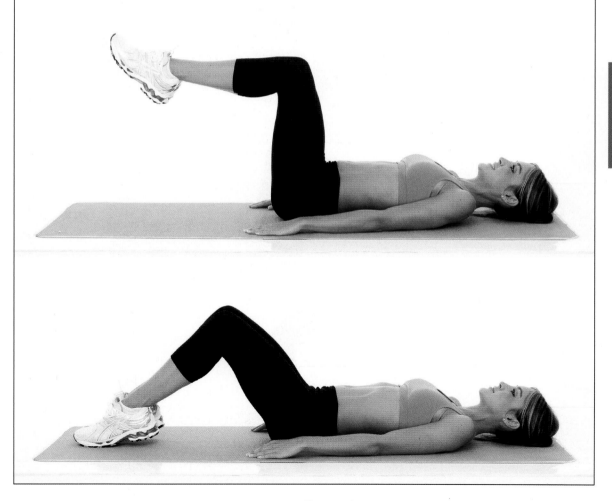

STRAIGHT-LEG CROSSOVER
Apple, boy, pear, hourglass

Areas trained: Upper stomach and side muscles
Technique:
★ Lie on your back and extend your legs up to the ceiling.
★ Crunch your shoulders up while reaching with your right hand towards your left foot.
★ Lower with control.
★ Crunch up, reaching with your left hand towards your right foot.
★ Repeat, alternating between left and right.

V-SIT

Apple, boy, pear, hourglass

Areas trained: All the stomach muscles
Technique:
★ Sit on the floor with your legs bent.
★ Keep your arms straight, next to your legs.
★ Lift both feet off the floor. This is the start position.
★ Extend your legs while simultaneously lowering your upper body towards the floor.
★ Bend your knees and lift your upper body back up to the start position.
★ Keeping your feet off the floor, repeat.

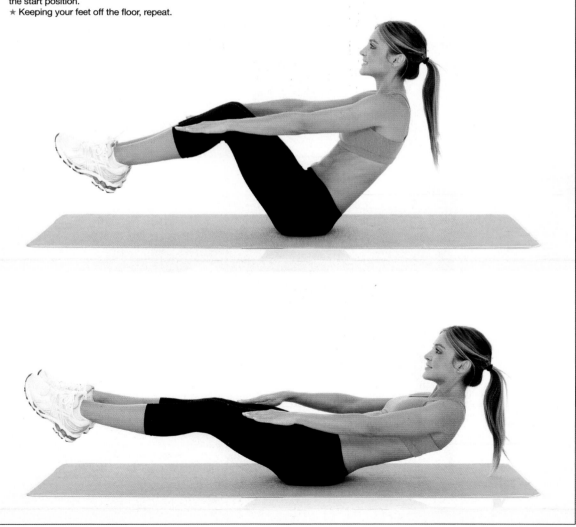

78

TWISTING V-SIT

Apple, boy, pear, hourglass

Areas trained: All stomach muscles
Technique:
★ Sit on the floor with your knees bent and your arms crossed over your chest.
★ Lift both feet off the floor. This is the start position.
★ Lower your upper body towards the floor while twisting your shoulders towards the right side, and extending your legs.
★ Lift up with control into the start position.
★ Repeat, twisting your shoulders towards the left side.
★ Alternate between left and right.

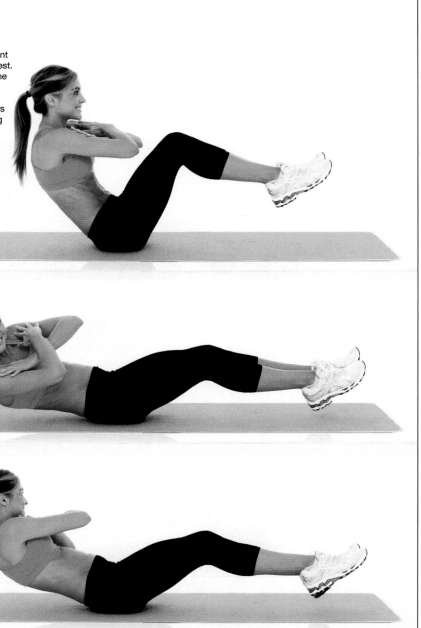

STRAIGHT-ARM CRUNCH
Apple, boy, pear, hourglass

Areas trained: Upper and lower stomach
Technique:
★ Lie on your back with your knees at a 90-degree angle.
★ Extend your right arm above your head and extend your right leg.
★ Keep your left leg at a 90-degree angle with your left hand behind your head.
★ Crunch your right arm and leg simultaneously up and reach towards your toes with your hand.
★ Lower with control.
★ Complete one set on the right side before repeating on the left.

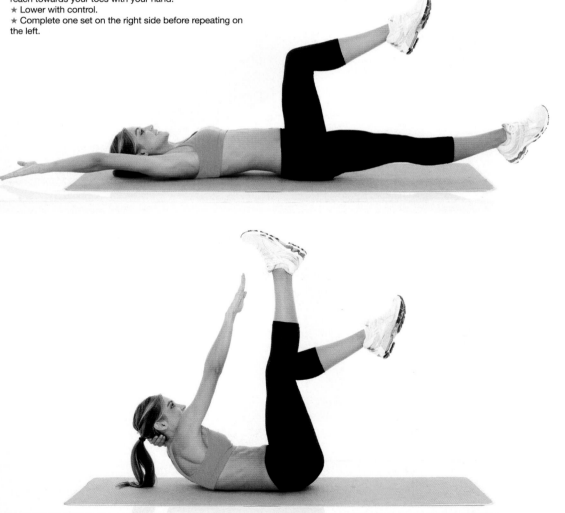

SLIDING BURPEE

Apple, boy, pear, hourglass

Area trained: Lower stomach
Technique:
★ You need a relatively slippery floor for this exercise.
★ Kneel on all fours.
★ Place your feet on a towel and your hands on the floor.
★ Lift your knees off the floor. This is the start position.
★ Pull your knees into your chest by sliding the towel forwards.
★ Push your feet backwards to the start position.
★ Keep your hands in the same position throughout the range of motion.

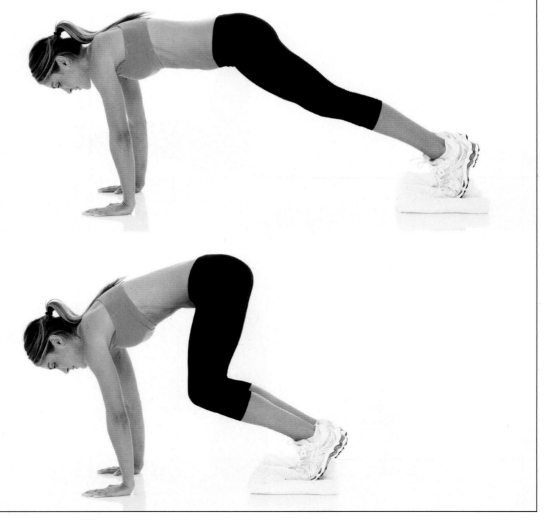

STABILITY BALL REVERSE CRUNCH

Apple, boy, pear, hourglass

Areas trained: Lower stomach and inner thighs
Technique:
★ Lie on your back and place your legs on a Stability Ball.
★ Tuck your heels into the ball and push it into your thighs.
★ Place your hands behind your head.
★ Crunch your upper body upwards while lifting the ball off the floor using your legs.
★ Lower, without allowing the ball to rest on the floor, and repeat.

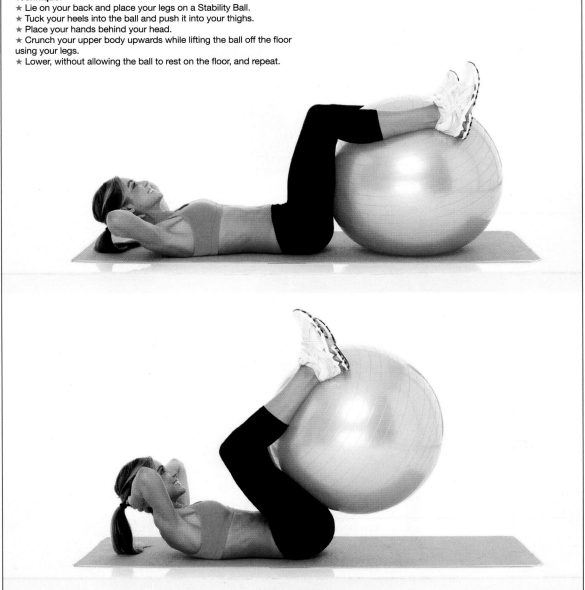

CYCLING
Apple, boy, pear, hourglass

Area trained: Lower stomach
Technique:
★ Lie on the floor with your knees bent, supporting your upper body with your elbows.
★ Keep your knees bent and lift your feet off the floor.
★ Extend your right leg while keeping the left leg bent.
★ Alternate between left and right to perform a cycling motion.

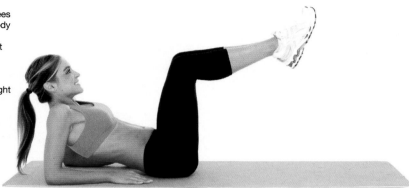

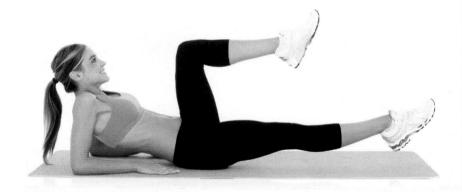

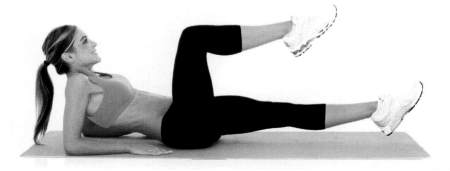

SCISSOR

Apple, boy, pear, hourglass

Area trained: Lower stomach
Technique:
★ Lie down on your back.
★ Put both hands behind your head and lift your head off the floor.
★ Keeping your legs straight, lift them off the floor at the same time.
★ Open your legs slightly wider than your hips.
★ Keeping your legs on the same level, close them, then repeat.
Tips:
★ Ensure that you keep your back flat on the floor.
★ The lower your legs are, the harder it will be.

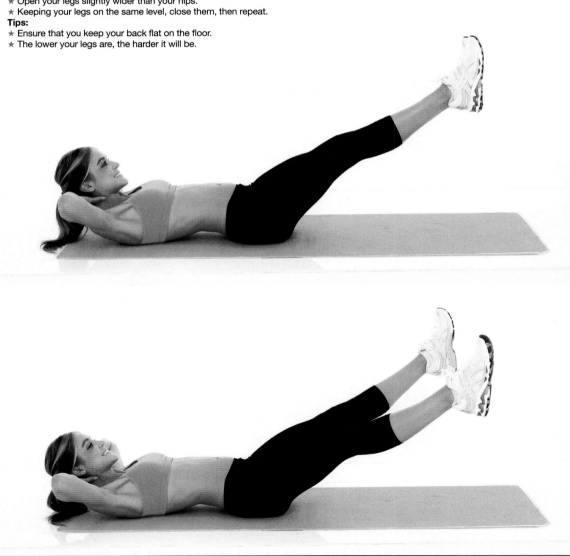

STABILITY BALL CRUNCH

Apple, boy, pear, hourglass

Areas trained: Core and upper stomach
Technique:
★ Lie with the small of your back supported by a Stability Ball.
★ Place your hands behind your head and look up.
★ Crunch your shoulders two inches off the ball, breathing out as you do so.
★ Lower with control, and repeat.
Tip:
★ Keep the movement small and it will be more effective.

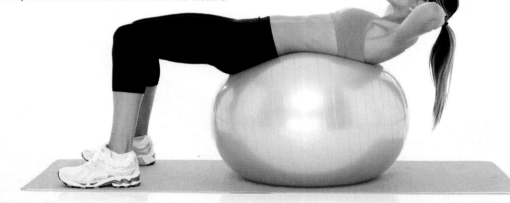

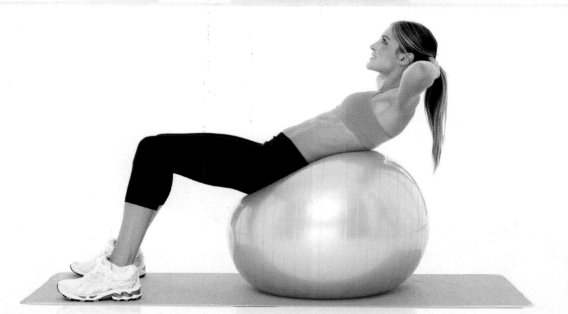

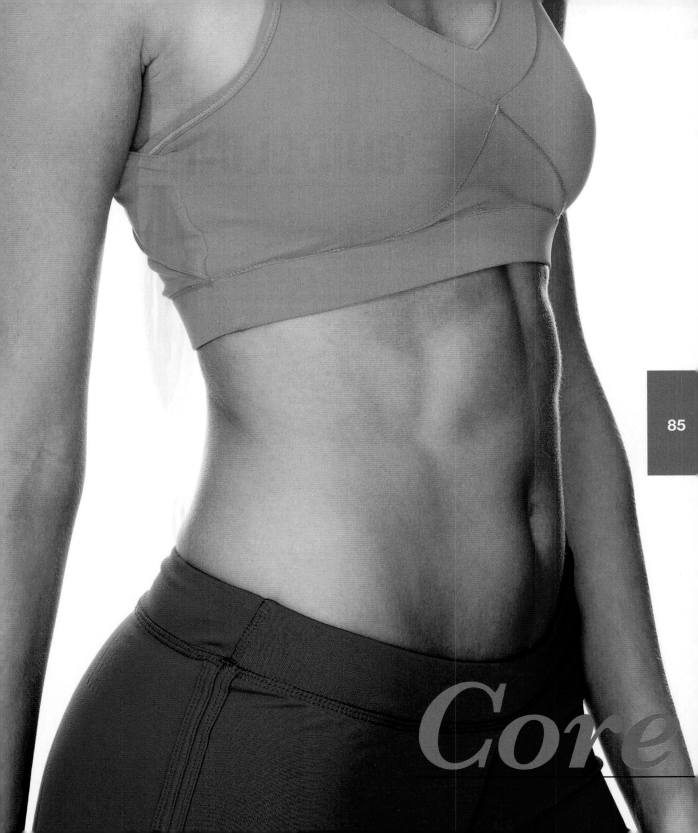

85

Core

CORE GUIDELINES

About the core

Your core muscles run the length of your torso, supporting your trunk and helping to keep your spine upright. Core stability, or the ability to control and co-ordinate the spine and pelvis during movement, is important because keeping the spine in a neutral position while exercising helps to prevent injuries. The stronger your core muscles, the more you'll get from your workout. Exercising the core is equally important for all bodyshapes.

APPLE

	REPS
BEGINNER	2 sets of 10 reps
INTERMEDIATE	2 sets of 15 reps
ADVANCED	2 sets of 20 reps

PEAR

	REPS
BEGINNER	2 sets of 10 reps
INTERMEDIATE	2 sets of 15 reps
ADVANCED	2 sets of 20 reps

HOURGLASS

	REPS
BEGINNER	2 sets of 10 reps
INTERMEDIATE	2 sets of 15 reps
ADVANCED	2 sets of 20 reps

BOY

	REPS
BEGINNER	2 sets of 10 reps
INTERMEDIATE	2 sets of 15 reps
ADVANCED	2 sets of 20 reps

ZIP-UP
Equally important for all bodyshapes

Areas trained: All the stomach and deeper back muscles
Technique:
★ Lie on the floor with your knees bent and your feet flat on the floor; don't tilt or tuck your pelvis.
★ Tense your stomach muscles by pulling your belly button towards your spine. Maintain a small natural arch in your lower back.
★ Hold the position for three breaths in and out before relaxing.

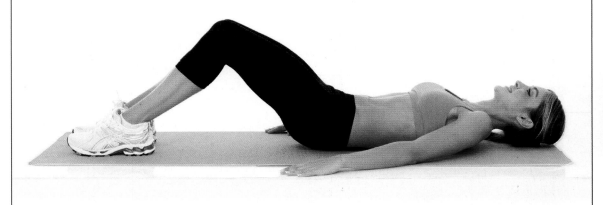

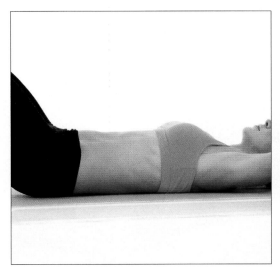

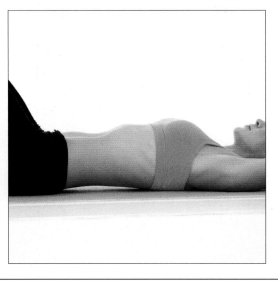

STRAIGHT LEG LOWERING

Equally important for all bodyshapes

Areas trained: All the stomach and deeper back muscles
Technique:
★ Lie on your back and extend both legs up to the ceiling.
★ Perform the zip-up move from this position (see previous exercise).
★ Lower your right leg down towards the floor.
★ If you feel your lower back arching, stop. Otherwise continue to lower your leg until your heel touches the floor.
★ Lift your right leg back up before repeating with the left leg.
★ Alternate between left and right.

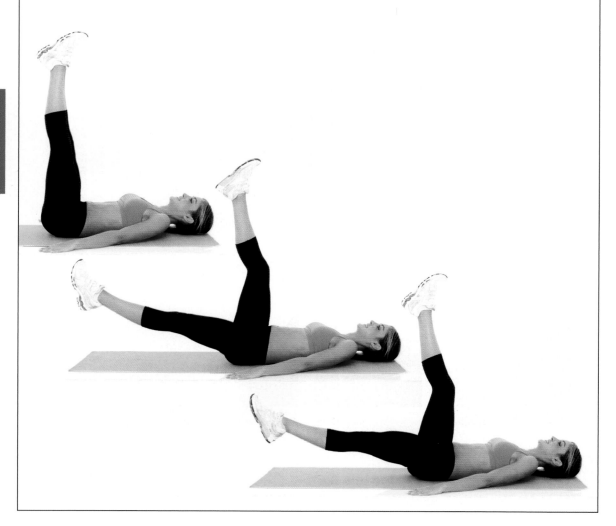

SPIDERMAN
Equally important for all bodyshapes

Areas trained: Core, stomach and arms

Technique:
★ Start in a push-up position with your hands level with your shoulders and your body in a straight line.
★ Lift your right foot off the floor and bring it in towards your right elbow.
★ Push your leg back and repeat on the left side.

Tip:
★ Aim to let your knee touch your elbow.

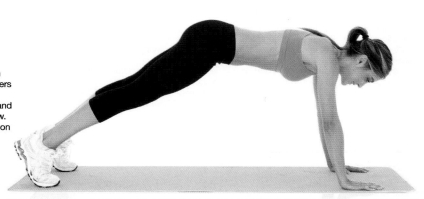

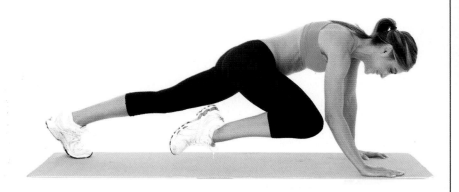

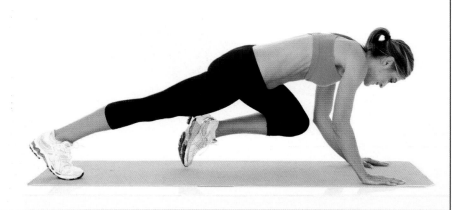

PLANK
Equally important for all bodyshapes

Areas trained: Core and stomach
Technique:
★ Lie on your stomach, resting your weight on your forearms, with your elbows underneath your shoulders.
★ Lift your body up on to your toes and elbows, keeping a straight line from your head to your heels, and being careful to keep your bottom down.
★ Beginners hold for 20–30 seconds for one set. Intermediates hold for 45-60 seconds for two sets with 30 seconds' rest between sets. Advanced hold for 60 seconds for three sets with 30 seconds' rest between sets.

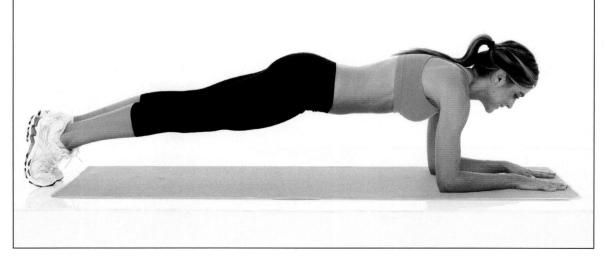

STABILITY BALL SIDE-TO-SIDE BRIDGE
Equally important for all bodyshapes

Areas trained: Core, stomach and legs
Technique:
★ Lie on your back with your feet on a Stability Ball and your arms by your sides.
★ Lift your hips off the floor so you have a straight line between your feet and your shoulders.
★ Roll both feet slightly over to the right side.
★ Return to the centre.
★ Roll over to the left side.
★ Alternate between right and left.

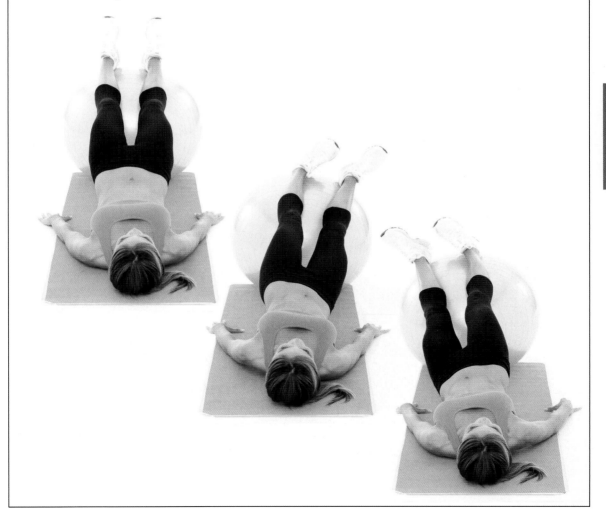

STABILITY BALL PLANK TWIST
Equally important for all bodyshapes

Area trained: Core and waist
Technique:
★ Kneel on all fours and place your feet on a Stability Ball, so your weight is on your hands and toes.
★ Keep your back straight and your belly button tight.
★ Roll the ball from left to right, twisting from your hips.

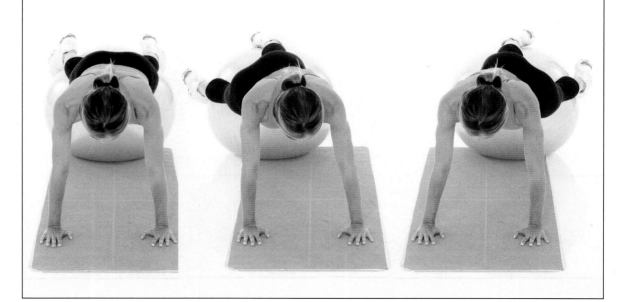

ROLLING PLANK
Equally important for all bodyshapes

Areas trained: Core and upper stomach
Technique:
★ Kneel behind a Stability Ball.
★ Put your elbows and forearms on the ball.
★ Ensure that your elbows are directly underneath your shoulders.
★ Lift your knees up so you are in a plank position (see page 90).
★ Roll the ball forward with your elbows.
★ Roll the ball back to the original position.
Tip:
★ Keep your hips in the same position throughout the range of motion.

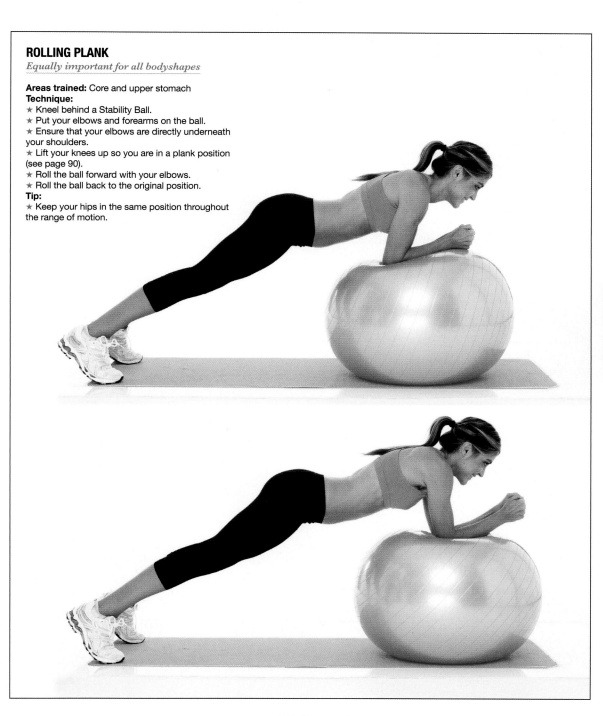

STABILITY BALL KNEE TUCK
Equally important for all bodyshapes

Areas trained: Core, thighs, stomach and arms
Technique:
★ Kneel on all fours, then place your feet up on a Stability Ball.
★ Ensure that you keep your back straight and your stomach tight.
This is the start position.
★ Roll the ball in towards your chest by bending your knees.
★ Push your bottom up towards the ceiling.
★ Straighten your body again, ensuring that you don't arch your back.

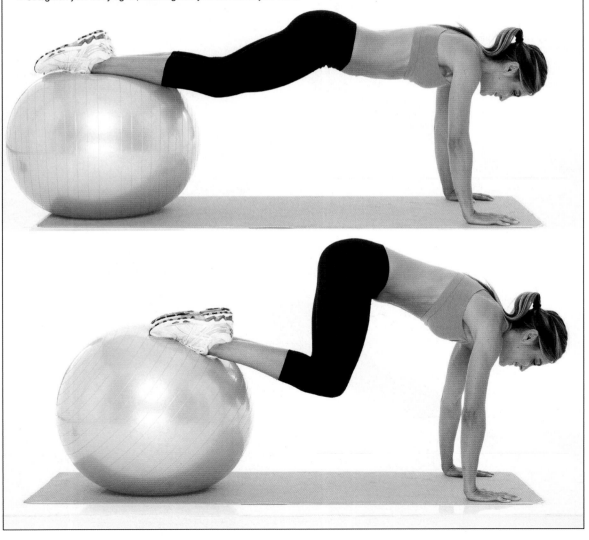

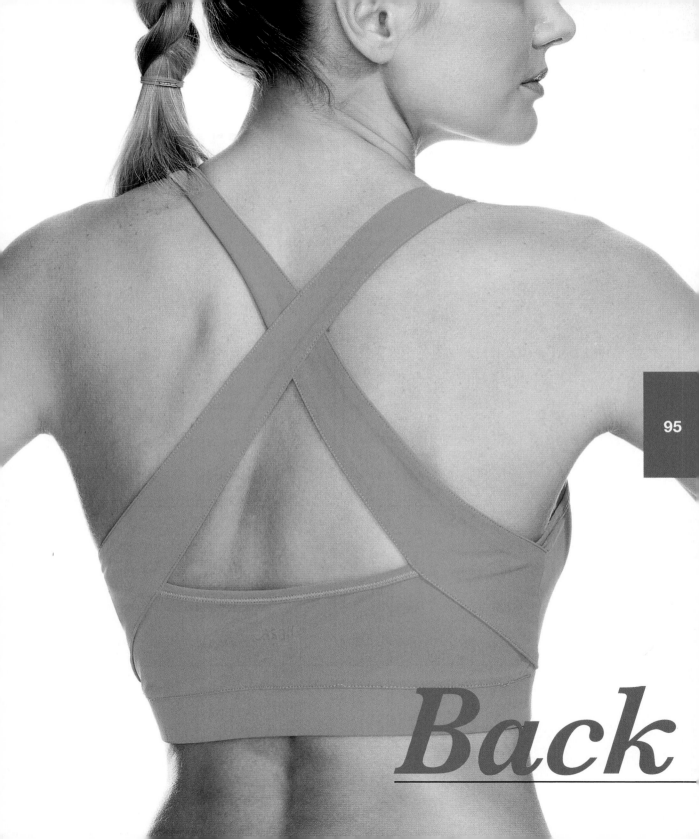

Back

BACK GUIDELINES

About the back

Your back can reveal a lot about your levels of bodyfat. If, when you look in the mirror, your bra digs in and bulges out across the back, then you should include at least two of these exercises in your workout. Apple and boy bodyshapes are particularly prone to storing fat on their backs.

Use a 2kg pair of dumbbells for all exercises that include weights

APPLE

	REPS
BEGINNER	2 sets of 15 reps
INTERMEDIATE	2 sets of 20 reps
ADVANCED	3 sets of 20 reps

PEAR

	REPS
BEGINNER	2 sets of 10 reps
INTERMEDIATE	2 sets of 15 reps
ADVANCED	2 sets of 20 reps

HOURGLASS

	REPS
BEGINNER	2 sets of 10 reps
INTERMEDIATE	2 sets of 15 reps
ADVANCED	2 sets of 20 reps

BOY

	REPS
BEGINNER	2 sets of 15 reps
INTERMEDIATE	2 sets of 20 reps
ADVANCED	3 sets of 20 reps

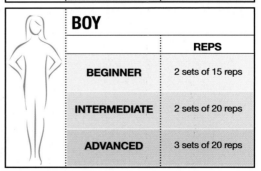

UNDER-GRIP BEND-OVER ROW

Apple, boy, pear, hourglass

Area trained: Upper back
Technique:
★ Stand with one foot in front of the other.
★ Hold a weight in each hand, with your palms facing up to the ceiling.
★ Bend your knees and lean forward with your upper body. This is the start position.
★ Pull your arms back, squeezing your shoulder blades together, so your hands are at waist level.
★ Extend your arms back to the start position and repeat.

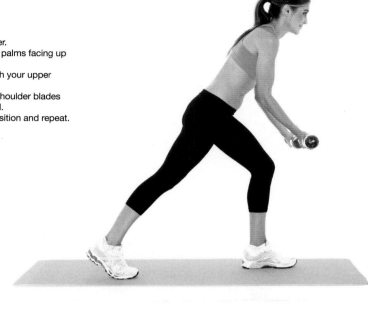

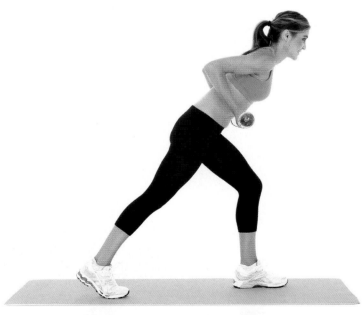

ELASTIC BAND ROW

Apple, boy, pear, hourglass

Area trained: Upper back

Technique:

★ Sit on the floor with your legs straight out in front of you.
★ Loop an elasticated band securely around your feet.
★ Grab hold of the band somewhere close to your feet.
★ Sit upright, so as to increase the resistance on the band.
★ Bend your arms and pull your hands towards your armpits.
★ Squeeze your shoulder blades together.
★ Slowly straighten out your arms and repeat.

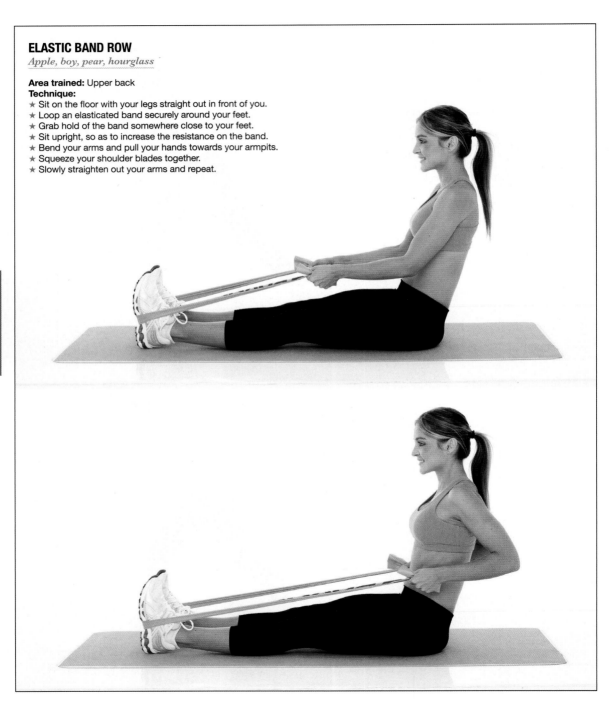

BALL BACK EXTENSION WITH SHOULDER SQUEEZE

Apple, boy, pear, hourglass

Area trained: Upper back

Technique:

★ Lie with your stomach on a Stability Ball.
★ Raise your arms so they are by your sides, palms facing up to the ceiling. This is the start position.
★ Lift your upper body, while turning your palms down to the floor.
★ Squeeze your shoulder blades.
★ Slowly lower and turn your palms back to the start position.

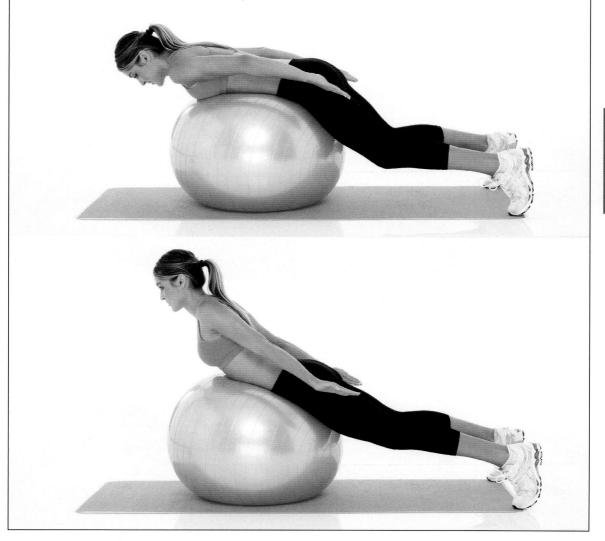

99

SUPERMAN

Apple, boy, pear, hourglass

Area trained: Lower back
Technique:
★ Lie on your stomach, with your arms stretched out in front of you.
★ Keeping your head on the floor, lift your left arm and your right leg into the air.
★ Hold the position for a second.
★ Lower and repeat with the right arm and left leg.
★ Alternate between left and right.

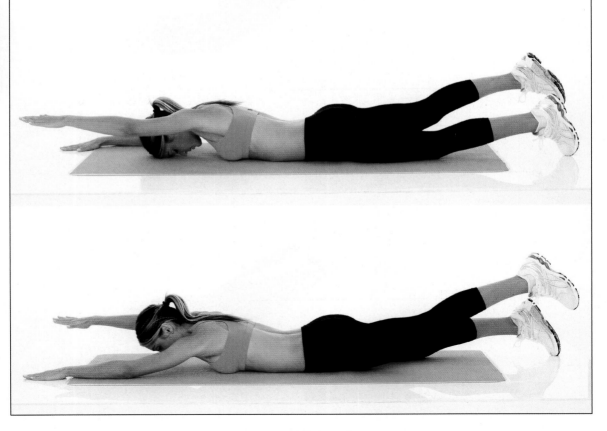

REVERSE STABILITY BALL BACK EXTENSION

Apple, boy, pear, hourglass

Area trained: Lower back
Technique:
★ Lie with your stomach on a Stability Ball, and your hands on the floor.
★ Keeping your legs straight, lift both of them off the floor.
★ Lift your legs until you have a straight line between your feet, knees, hips and shoulders.
★ Your spine should be in a neutral (natural) position at this point. Hold the position for one to two seconds.
★ Lower your legs with control, until your feet touch the floor.
Tips:
★ Don't bounce on the ball.
★ Breathe out when lifting your legs.

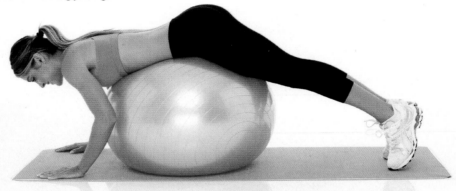

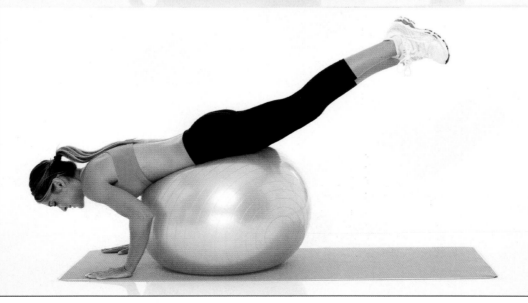

QL LIFTS

Apple, boy, pear, hourglass

Area trained: Lower back
Technique:
★ Lie on your stomach.
★ Lift your right leg off the floor without rolling your hips.
★ Move your right leg sideways.
★ Move your leg back in and lower it, but don't rest it on the floor.
★ Complete one set before repeating with the left leg.

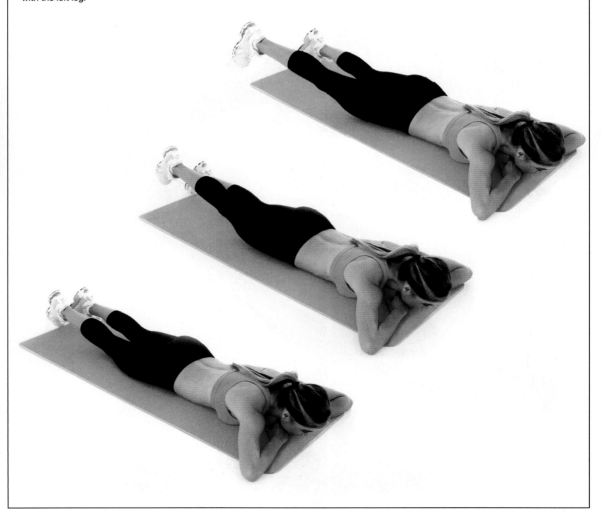

102

SINGLE ARM ROW

Apple, boy, pear, hourglass

Areas trained: Triceps, back and shoulders

Technique:

★ Stand with your right foot in front of your left, holding a weight in your left hand, with your palm facing in.

★ Lean forward from the waist and support yourself on a chair, or on your right thigh, with your right hand.

★ Let your left arm with the weight hang down. This is the start position.

★ Ensure that your back is flat.

★ Lift the weight up towards your waist, pulling your arm back and squeezing your shoulder blade.

★ Slowly lower the weight back to the start position and repeat.

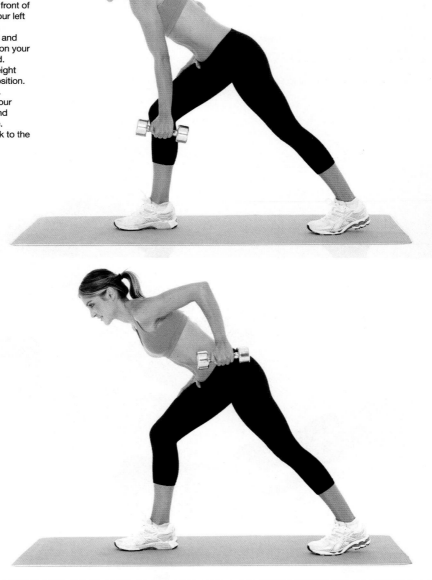

104

BACK EXTENSION WITH SIDE BEND

Apple, boy, pear, hourglass

Area trained: Lower back
Technique:
★ Lie on your stomach.
★ Keep your arms by your sides, palms facing upwards.
★ Lift your upper body off the floor.
★ Bend sideways towards the left.
★ Return to the centre position and lower your body.
★ Repeat towards the right side.
★ Alternate between left and right.
Tip:
★ Keep your feet on the floor at all times.

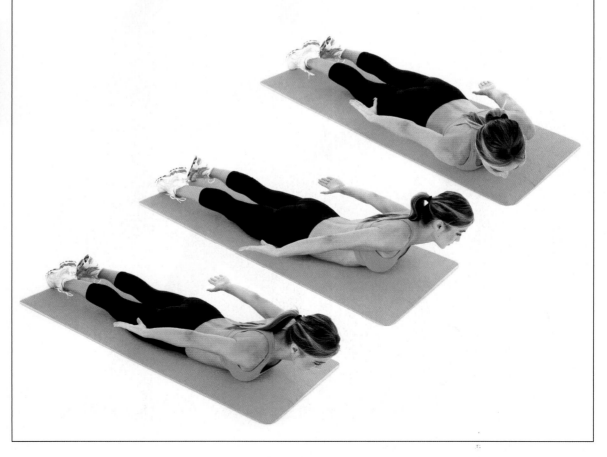

bottom

BOTTOM GUIDELINES

About the bottom

Exercising the bottom is particularly important for hourglass and pear bodyshapes, as they will find it hardest to shift weight from this area. If this includes you, incorporate at least two of the following exercises into your bodyshape workout.

Use a 2kg pair of dumbbells for all exercises that include weights

APPLE

	REPS
BEGINNER	2 sets of 10 reps
INTERMEDIATE	2 sets of 15 reps
ADVANCED	2 sets of 20 reps

PEAR

	REPS
BEGINNER	2 sets of 15 reps
INTERMEDIATE	2 sets of 20 reps
ADVANCED	3 sets of 20 reps

HOURGLASS

	REPS
BEGINNER	2 sets of 15 reps
INTERMEDIATE	2 sets of 20 reps
ADVANCED	3 sets of 20 reps

BOY

	REPS
BEGINNER	2 sets of 10 reps
INTERMEDIATE	2 sets of 15 reps
ADVANCED	2 sets of 20 reps

106

GLUTE LIFT WITH PULSES

Hourglass, pear, boy, apple

Area trained: Bottom
Technique:

★ Kneel on all fours.
★ Lift your left knee off the floor and flex your left foot.
★ Lift your left knee up until it's level with your hip.
★ Lower with control.
★ Complete one set and then hold the top position.
★ Pulse by lifting your knee about one to two inches higher for a second, then lowering it back to the top position.
★ Complete the same number of pulses as you did reps, before moving on to the right leg.

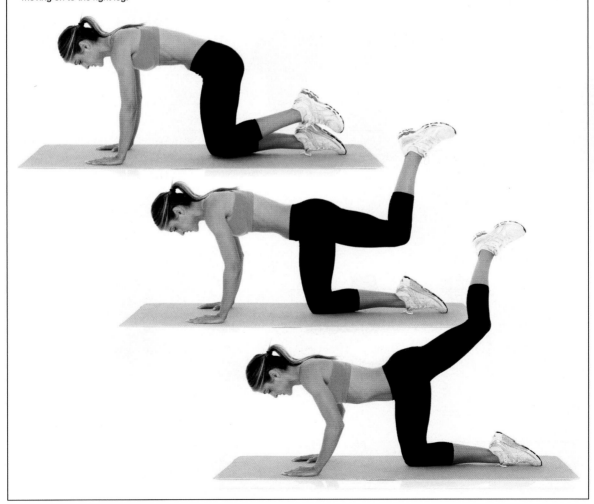

107

STABILITY BALL GLUTE LIFT
Hourglass, pear, boy, apple

Area trained: Bottom
Technique:
★ Place your hands on the floor and rest your lower legs on a Stability Ball.
★ Take your right leg off the ball, keeping your knee bent.
★ Push your right heel up to the ceiling and squeeze your bottom.
★ Lower your right leg.
★ Complete one set before repeating with your left leg.
Tip:
★ If you feel pain in your lower back your hips are too low, so lift your bottom higher.

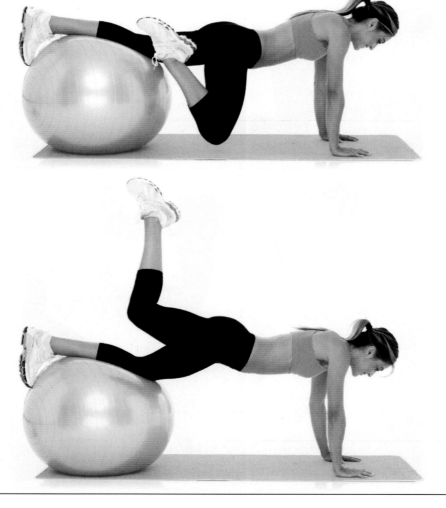

108

LUNGE STEP-UP

Hourglass, pear, boy, apple

Areas trained: Thighs and bottom
Technique:
★ Stand behind a step, holding a weight in each hand.
★ Place your left foot on the step.
★ Bend both knees, lowering your right knee to the floor.
★ Push up and place your right foot on the step.
★ Step backwards off the step with both legs.
★ Repeat with your right leg.
★ Alternate between your left and right leg.

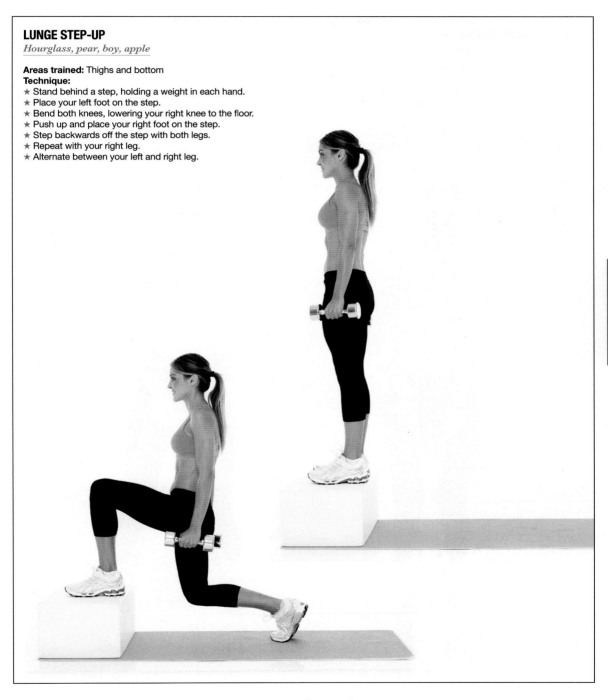

109

ELASTIC BAND CRAB WALK

Hourglass, pear, boy, apple

Areas trained: Bottom and outer thighs
Technique:
★ Stand with both feet on an elasticated band.
★ Cross the band in front of your legs and hold on to the handles.
★ Keeping your back straight and your shoulders well back, take one step sideways, keeping your legs straight.
★ Bring your feet back together and step towards the other side.
★ Keep alternating from side to side for set number of reps.

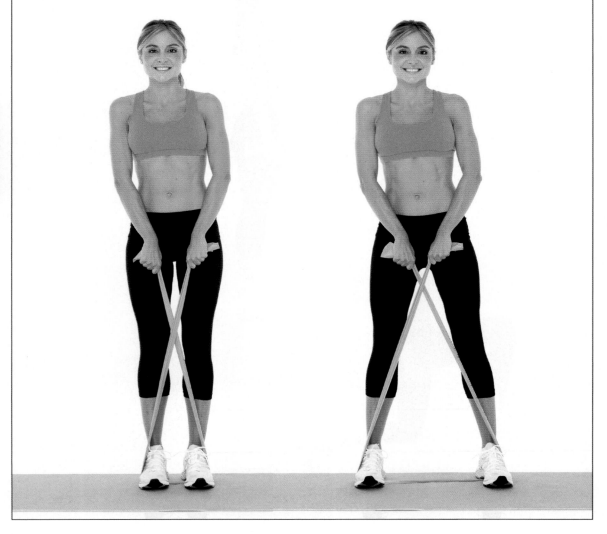

SINGLE-LEG BRIDGE

Hourglass, pear, boy, apple

Area trained: Bottom
Technique:
★ Lie on your back with your feet on a Stability Ball and your arms by your sides.
★ Extend your left leg up to the ceiling.
★ Keep your right heel on the ball and your leg straight.
★ Lift your bottom off the floor, ensuring that you keep your hips level.
★ Roll the ball towards you with your right foot, lifting your hips towards the ceiling as you do so.
★ Hold the top position for a second.
★ Lower but don't rest your bottom on the floor.
★ Complete one set before repeating on the other side.

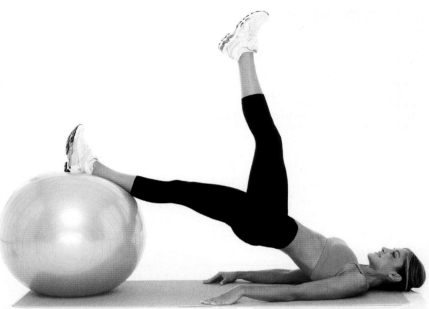

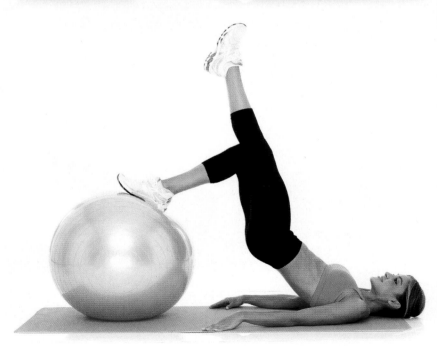

111

LYING 45-DEGREE LEG LIFT

Hourglass, pear, boy, apple

Area trained: Bottom
Technique:
★ Lie on your right side and extend your left leg out in front of you at an angle of about 45 degrees.
★ Keeping your left leg straight, and your toes facing down, lift it off the floor up to about hip height.
★ Lower your leg until your toes touch the floor again.
★ Complete one set before repeating on the other side.

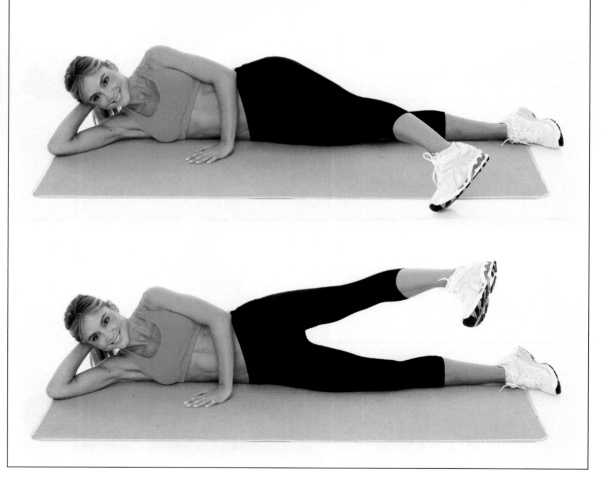

STANDING SIDE-KICK

Hourglass, pear, boy, apple

Area trained: Bottom

Technique:

★ Place all your bodyweight on your left leg and lean over to the left.
★ Lift your right leg sideways until it's level with your hip.
★ Bend your right knee and kick your leg out.
★ Complete one set on the left leg before changing to the right leg.

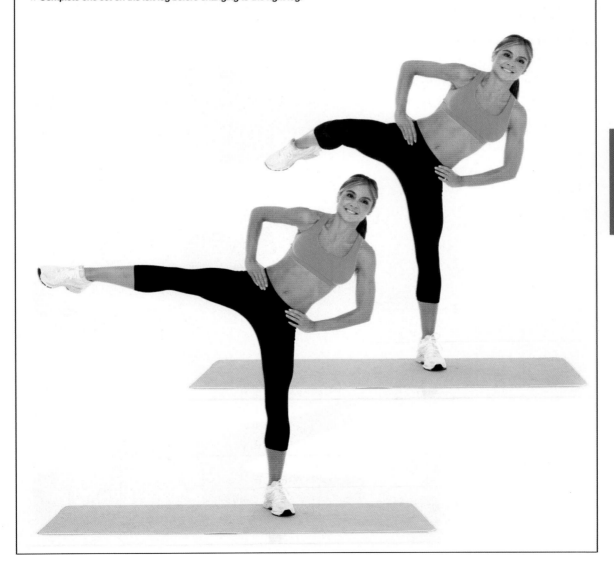

113

LYING SIDE LEG LIFT AND EXTENSION

Hourglass, pear, boy, apple

Area trained: Bottom
Technique:
★ Lie on your left side and place your right leg at a 90-degree angle on the floor in front of you. This is the start position.
★ Lift your right leg up to hip height with your knee still bent.
★ Extend your leg, keeping it slightly higher than your hip.
★ Return to the start position by reversing the move.
★ Complete one set with your right leg before repeating with your left.
Tip:
★ Don't let your knee rest on the floor.

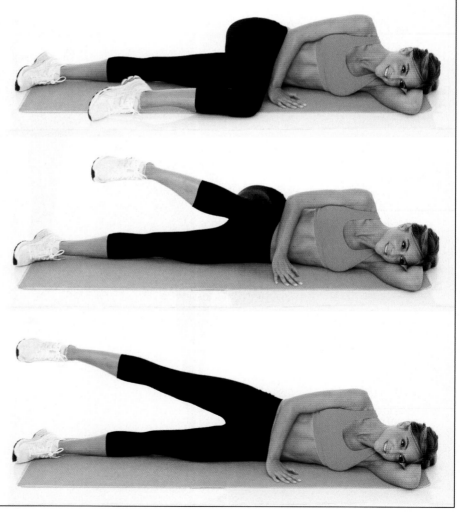

114

STEP BOTTOM EXTENSION
Hourglass, pear, boy, apple

Area trained: Bottom
Technique:
★ Stand with your right leg on a step, and extend your left leg backwards.
★ Bend your right knee and push your left leg further back.
★ Squeeze your bottom.
★ Keep your tummy tight throughout the range of motion.
★ Repeat the exercise on the right leg before switching to the left.

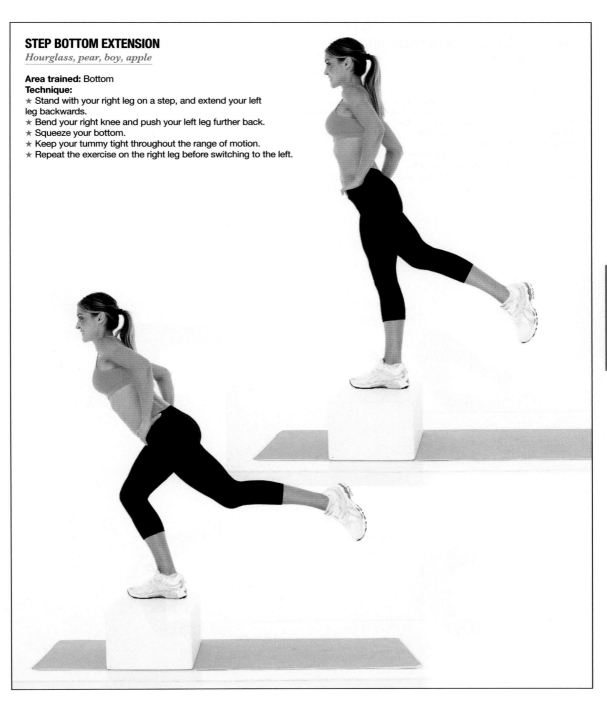

115

STABILITY BALL SIDE LEG LIFT WITH ROTATIONS
Hourglass, pear, boy, apple

Area trained: Bottom
Technique:
★ Kneel on the floor beside a Stability Ball.
★ Lean with your left side over the ball and extend your right leg sideways.
★ Lift your right leg off the floor until it is level with your hip.
★ Hold the top position and rotate your leg in a circular movement clockwise before lowering your leg.
★ Repeat the move but this time rotate your leg anticlockwise.
★ Only do one rotation for each repetition.
★ Complete one set with your right leg before repeating with your left.

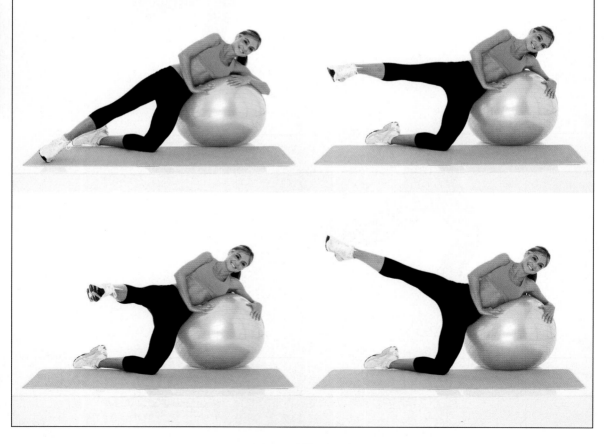

Legs

LEGS GUIDELINES

About the legs

Pear and hourglass bodyshapes store most of their bodyfat around their legs and thighs. Toning your legs is a very important aid to inch-loss. Do at least four exercises every time you work out: one for your inner thighs, one for your outer thighs, one for the front of your thighs and one for the back. If you would like more defined ankles, you should also include the Stability Ball seated calf raises on page 128 in your workout.

Use a 2kg pair of dumbbells for all exercises that include weights

APPLE

	REPS
BEGINNER	2 sets of 10 reps
INTERMEDIATE	2 sets of 15 reps
ADVANCED	2 sets of 20 reps

PEAR

	REPS
BEGINNER	2 sets of 15 reps
INTERMEDIATE	2 sets of 20 reps
ADVANCED	3 sets of 20 reps

HOURGLASS

	REPS
BEGINNER	2 sets of 15 reps
INTERMEDIATE	2 sets of 20 reps
ADVANCED	3 sets of 20 reps

BOY

	REPS
BEGINNER	2 sets of 10 reps
INTERMEDIATE	2 sets of 15 reps
ADVANCED	2 sets of 20 reps

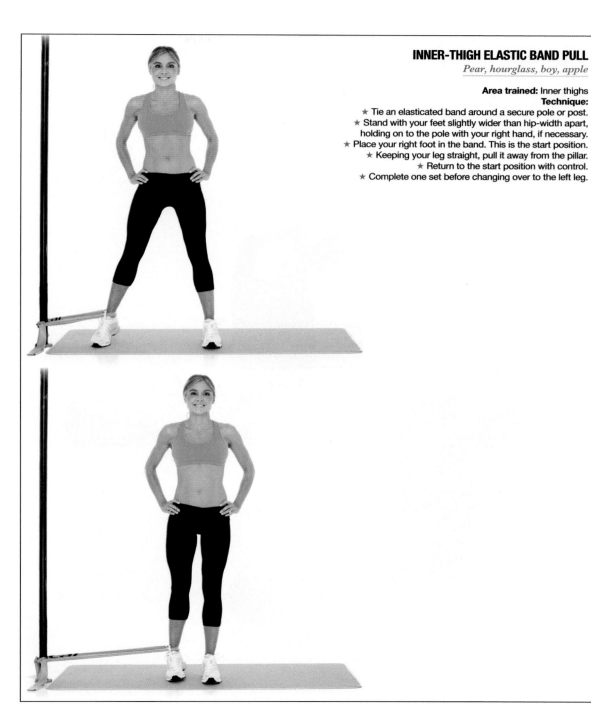

INNER-THIGH ELASTIC BAND PULL
Pear, hourglass, boy, apple

Area trained: Inner thighs
Technique:
★ Tie an elasticated band around a secure pole or post.
★ Stand with your feet slightly wider than hip-width apart,
holding on to the pole with your right hand, if necessary.
★ Place your right foot in the band. This is the start position.
★ Keeping your leg straight, pull it away from the pillar.
★ Return to the start position with control.
★ Complete one set before changing over to the left leg.

119

BALL SQUEEZE
Pear, hourglass, boy, apple

Area trained: Inner thighs
Technique:
★ Lie on your back with your knees bent and place a Medicine ball between your knees.
★ Lift your feet off the floor to create a right angle at your hips.
★ Squeeze your knees together and hold for two seconds.
★ Relax but keep your legs in the same position with the ball between your knees.

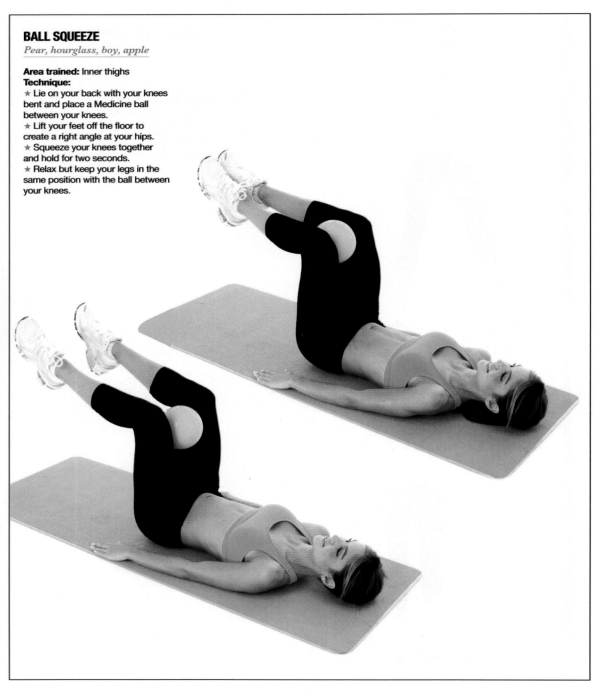

WIDE PULSING SQUATS

Pear, hourglass, boy, apple

Areas trained: Inner and front thighs
Technique:
★ Stand with your feet about twice your shoulder-width apart.
★ Turn your toes out at a 45-degree angle.
★ Bend your knees until you have a 90-degree angle at your hips and knees. This is the start position.
★ Lift yourself up a few inches then lower back to the start position and repeat.

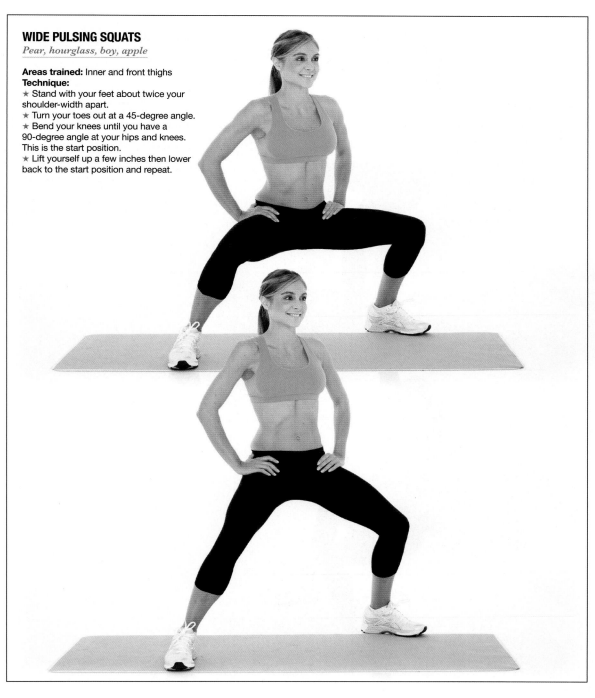

121

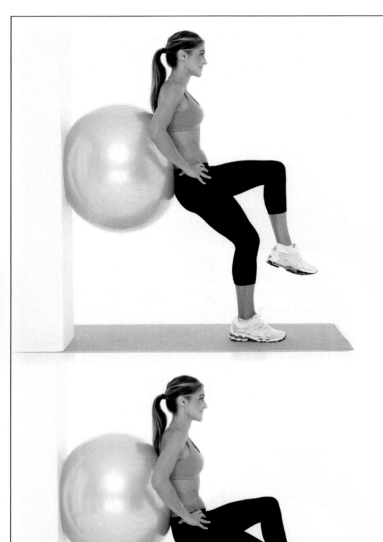

STABILITY BALL SINGLE-LEG SQUAT
Pear, hourglass, boy, apple

Areas trained: Front thighs and balance
Technique:
★ Stand against a wall with your lower back supported by a Stability Ball.
★ Keep your right foot in line with your belly button and lift your left foot off the floor. This is the start position.
★ Bend your right knee and lower your bottom to the floor.
★ Go as low as you can while remaining in control of the movement.
★ Push back up to the start position.
★ Repeat one set on your right leg before changing over to your left leg.

122

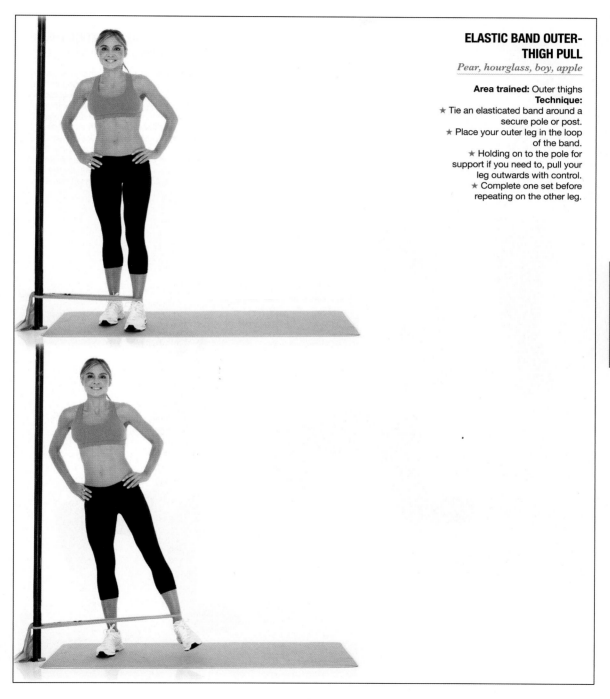

ELASTIC BAND OUTER-THIGH PULL
Pear, hourglass, boy, apple

Area trained: Outer thighs
Technique:
★ Tie an elasticated band around a secure pole or post.
★ Place your outer leg in the loop of the band.
★ Holding on to the pole for support if you need to, pull your leg outwards with control.
★ Complete one set before repeating on the other leg.

123

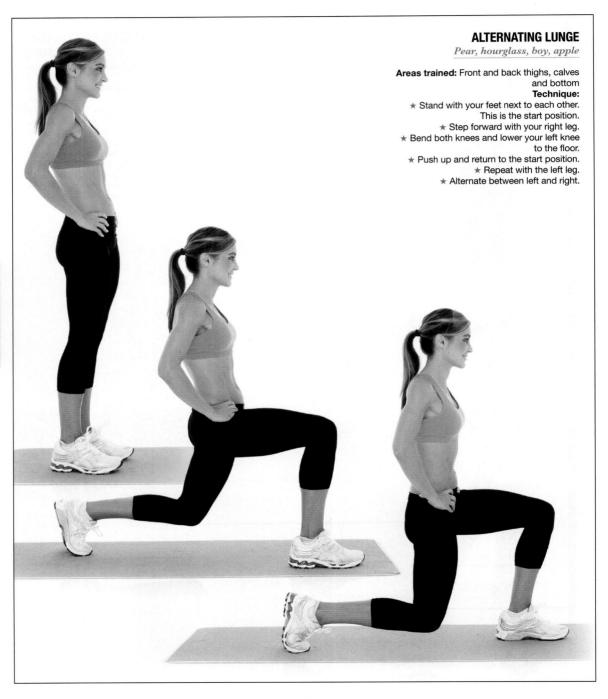

ALTERNATING LUNGE
Pear, hourglass, boy, apple

Areas trained: Front and back thighs, calves and bottom
Technique:
★ Stand with your feet next to each other. This is the start position.
★ Step forward with your right leg.
★ Bend both knees and lower your left knee to the floor.
★ Push up and return to the start position.
★ Repeat with the left leg.
★ Alternate between left and right.

124

STABILITY BALL LUNGE

Pear, hourglass, boy, apple

Areas trained: Thighs, hips, balance and coordination

Technique:

★ Stand in front of a Stability Ball with your knees together, and place your left foot on the ball.

★ Bend your right knee and roll the ball backwards with your left foot.

★ Stand back up and roll the ball forwards until your knees are together again.

★ Repeat one set on your right leg before changing to the left leg.

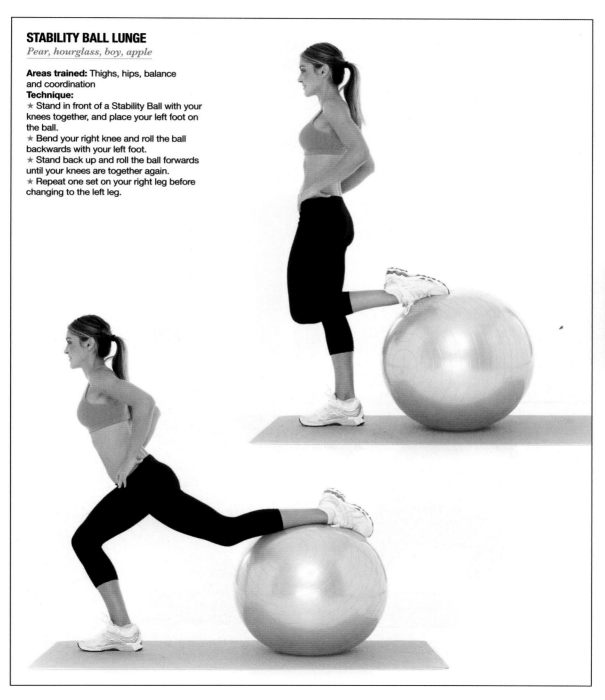

125

DIAGONAL LUNGE OFF A STEP
Pear, hourglass, boy, apple

Areas trained: Front, back and inner thighs
Technique:

★ Stand on a Step with your feet shoulder-width apart.
★ With your hands on your hips, take a big step forward off the Step with your right leg, placing your right foot on the floor.
★ Keeping your hips facing forward, bend both knees to perform a lunge.
★ Push back on to the Step, squeezing your bottom when stepping back to help your balance.
★ Repeat with the left leg.
★ Alternate between left and right.

126

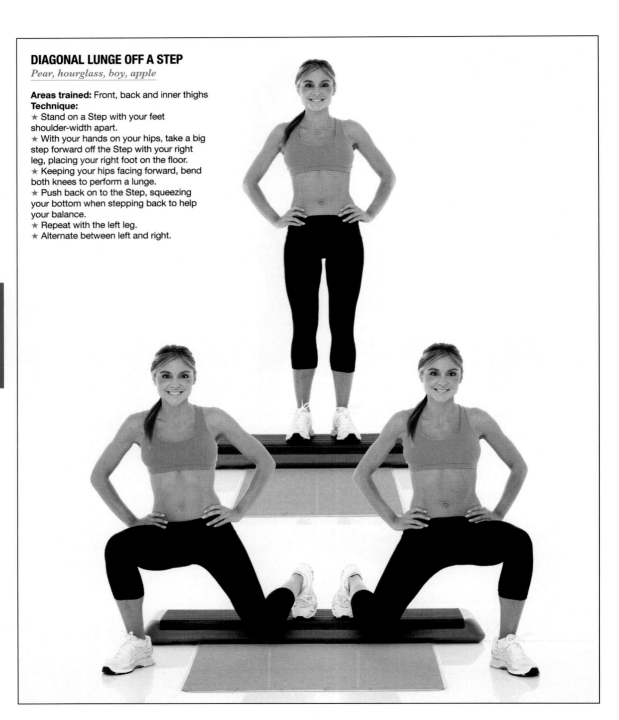

STABILITY BALL LEG CURL

Pear, hourglass, boy, apple

Area trained: Back of thighs
Technique:
★ Lie on your back with your heels on a Stability Ball.
★ Keeping your arms on the floor next to your body, lift your bottom off the floor. This is the start position.
★ Bend your knees and pull them up towards your chest.
★ Don't drop your hips down.
★ Extend your legs back to the start position and repeat.

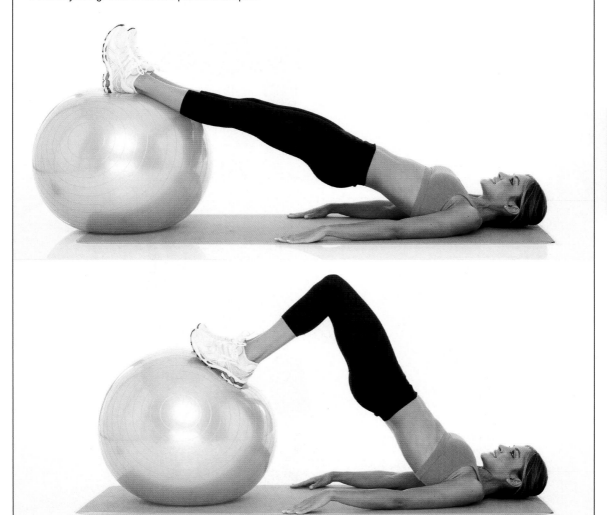

127

STABILITY BALL SEATED CALF RAISE
Pear, hourglass, boy, apple

Area trained: Calves
Technique:
★ Sit on a Stability Ball, holding a weight on each knee.
★ Lift up on to your toes.
★ Slowly lower your feet until your heels touch the floor again and repeat.

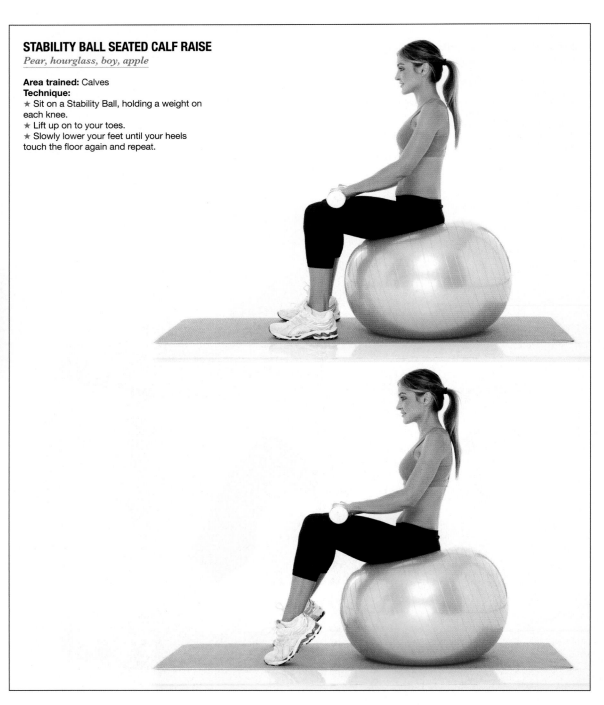

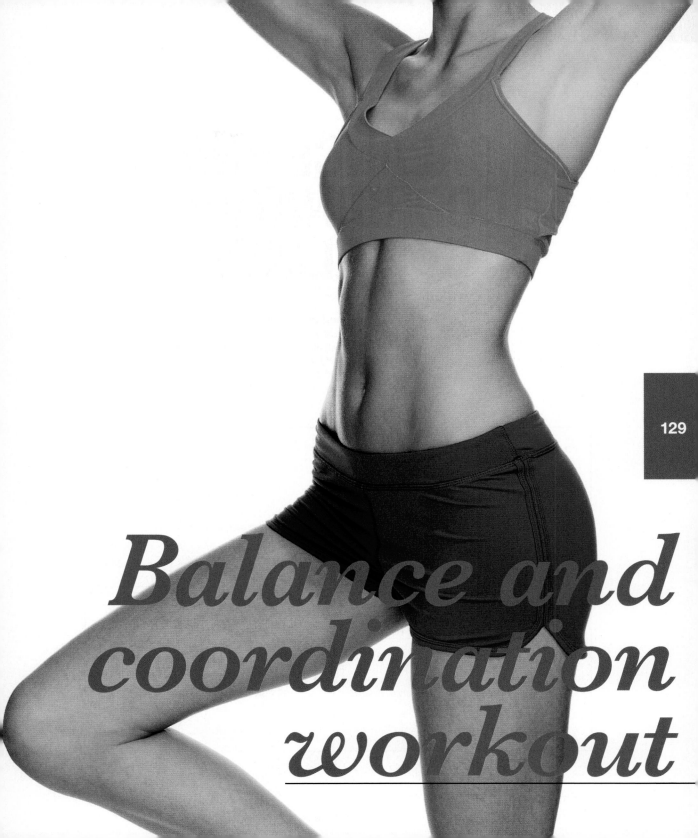

Balance and coordination workout

BALANCE AND COORDINATION GUIDELINES

About balance and coordination

Good balance and coordination are important for all bodyshapes. When you work on these, you will also improve the connection between your brain and muscles, which helps your body to function more effectively, and reduces your risk of injury. In addition, enhanced balance and coordination will give your cardiovascular performance a boost.

130

APPLE

	REPS
BEGINNER	1 set of 10 reps
INTERMEDIATE	2 sets of 10 reps
ADVANCED	3 sets of 10 reps

PEAR

	REPS
BEGINNER	1 set of 10 reps
INTERMEDIATE	2 sets of 10 reps
ADVANCED	3 sets of 10 reps

HOURGLASS

	REPS
BEGINNER	1 set of 10 reps
INTERMEDIATE	2 sets of 10 reps
ADVANCED	3 sets of 10 reps

BOY

	REPS
BEGINNER	1 set of 10 reps
INTERMEDIATE	2 sets of 10 reps
ADVANCED	3 sets of 10 reps

FLAMINGO
Equally important for all bodyshapes

Areas trained: Core, balance
and coordination
Technique:
★ Stand on your right leg and lift your left
leg off the floor.
★ Keep your eyes closed for 20 seconds at
first, working up to one minute. Relax and
repeat for set number of reps.
★ Use your arms for balance but don't hold
on to anything. Repeat on your left leg.

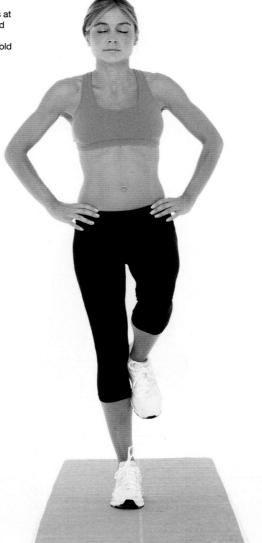

131

KNEELING ON A STABILITY BALL
Equally important for all bodyshapes

Areas trained: Core, balance and coordination
Technique:
★ Stand behind a Stability Ball.
★ Place your hands and knees on the ball.
★ Roll the ball forward.
★ Lift your hands off the ball.
★ Balance for 5-10 seconds, relax and repeat for set number of reps.
Tip:
★ Ensure that there is enough space to perform this exercise!

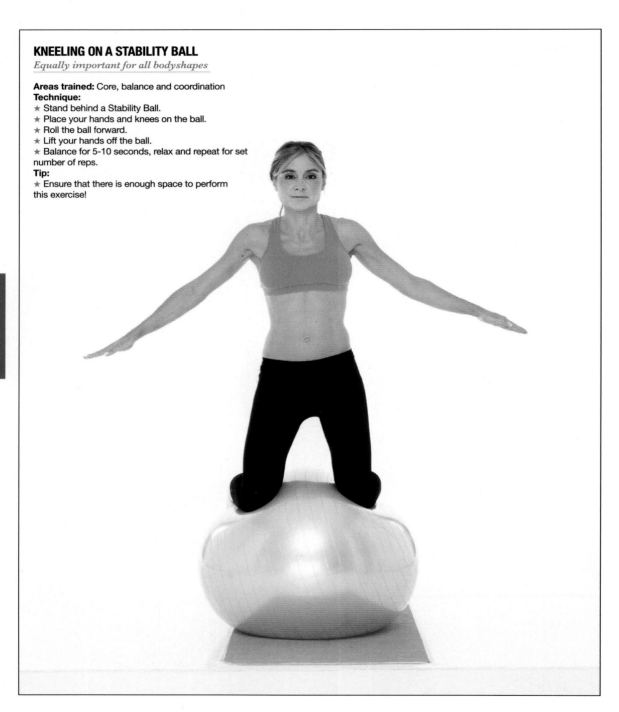

132

STABILITY BALL BRIDGE WITH ARMS CROSSED
Equally important for all bodyshapes

Areas trained: Core, balance and coordination
Technique:
★ Lie on your back with your feet on a Stability Ball and your arms crossed over your chest.
★ Lift your hips off the floor so you have a straight line between your feet and your shoulders.
★ Keep your tummy tight and squeeze your bottom.
★ Hold the position for five seconds, relax and repeat for set number of reps.

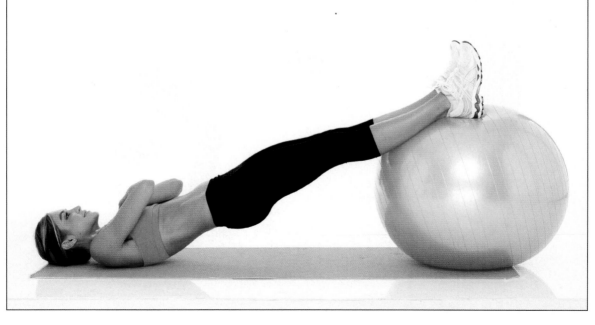

WOODCHOP
Equally important for all bodyshapes

Areas trained: Core, balance and coordination

Technique:

★ Stand on your right leg. Extend your left arm up to the ceiling and your left leg out behind you. This is the start position.

★ Bend your right knee, taking your left hand down and touching a point just to the outside of your right calf.

★ Return to the start position. Complete set number of reps and repeat on other side.

134

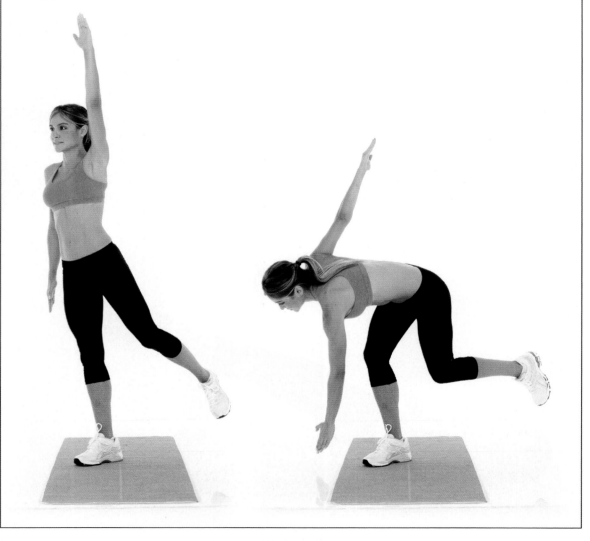

STAR STANCE
Equally important for all bodyshapes

Areas trained: Core, balance and coordination
Technique:
★ Stand up tall and place all your bodyweight on your left leg.
★ Spread your arms sideways. This is the start position.
★ Lift your right leg sideways off the floor to form a five-pointed star, with your left arm pointing towards the floor.
★ Hold the position for five seconds.
★ Return to the start position. Complete set number of reps and repeat on other side.
Tip:
★ If you find this difficult at first, try doing it with your back against a wall.

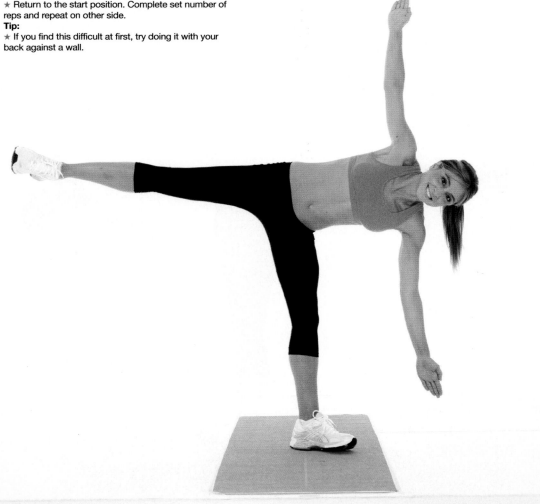

135

T-STANCE
Equally important for all bodyshapes

Areas trained: Core, balance and coordination
Technique:
★ Stand up tall and place all your bodyweight on your right leg.
★ Extend your left leg backwards and your arms sideways. This is the start position.
★ Pivot your upper body forwards, and your left leg backwards.
★ Aim for a straight line between your head, right hip and left foot.
★ Hold the position for five seconds.
★ Return to the start position. Complete set number of reps and repeat on other side.

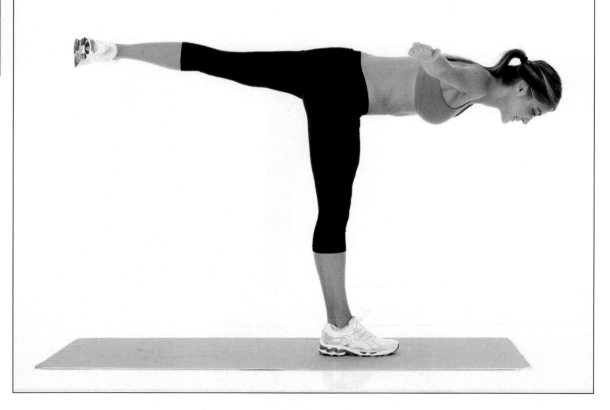

Nutrition

★ **Hourglass diet**
★ **Boy diet**
★ **Apple diet**
★ **Pear diet**

There are four weeks' worth of meal ideas for each bodyshape. Simply choose a breakfast, lunch and dinner each day from your bodyshape meal plan for a varied and filling diet to complement your bodyshape and fitness regime. The tailored plans will also help you lose up to half a stone in four weeks when combined with the cardio plans and toning exercises.

HOURGLASS

Hourglass shapes tend to be tempted by saturated fats, like the crisp fat on certain cuts of meat, and sugary foods. Choose lean meat including skinless chicken, fish, eggs, fresh fruit and vegetables. Avoid cooked, high-GI vegetables, such as carrots, parsnips and potatoes, and steer clear of fizzy drinks and sugar-rich foodstuffs.

BREAKFAST

■ Natural yoghurt, fruit and toasted sunflower seeds
Cut up three of your favourite fruits (e.g. a pear, a couple of plums and a few raspberries) and mix with 2tsps of low-fat natural yoghurt. Sprinkle with toasted sunflower seeds.

cals 226 | fat 2.5g | sat fat 0.5g | protein 12g

■ Ham and scrambled eggs
Scramble two eggs with a dash of skimmed milk and season to taste. Serve with 2 slices of lean ham.

cals 262 | fat 16.3g | sat fat 3.5g | protein 25g

■ Cereal with fruit and nuts
Mix together 40g of bran flakes or All Bran with 2-3 chopped dried apricots and 1tsp of chopped toasted walnuts. Serve with 125ml of semi-skimmed milk.

cals 289 | fat 4g | sat fat 2g | protein 10g

■ Porridge and natural yoghurt
Make a bowl of porridge in the microwave or on the hob with 40g of oats (not powdered) and semi-skimmed milk according to packet instructions. Serve with 1tbsp of low-fat natural yoghurt in the middle.

cals 248 | fat 4.7g | sat fat 0.7g | protein 5.9g

■ Grilled mushrooms and poached egg on toast
Grill 2 large Portobello mushrooms and serve on top of 1 slice of wholemeal toast with 1 poached egg on top.

cals 223 | fat 15.6g | sat fat 3.9g | protein 11.7g

■ Muesli with grated apple and toasted nuts
A bowl of sugar-free muesli (50g) with 1 peeled grated apple, 1tbsp of toasted chopped hazelnuts and 125ml of semi-skimmed milk.

cals 353 | fat 5.5g | sat fat 1.8g | protein 12g

■ Smoked salmon and scrambled eggs
Scramble 2 eggs in a pan with 1tsp of butter and serve with 25g of smoked salmon cut into thin strips, and snipped chives if desired.

cals 234 | fat 8.6g | sat fat 1.7g | protein 8.9g

■ Wholemeal muffin
Toast 1 wholemeal muffin, cut in half and spread with Flora Light.

cals 145 | fat 3.5g | sat fat 1g | protein 8g

■ Breakfast fruit smoothie
Make a smoothie from 1 small ripe banana, 1 apple and 140g of blueberries. Process until smooth, and add some apple juice to dilute. Stir in a little honey to taste, and serve.

cals 124 | fat 0g | sat fat 0g | protein 3g

■ Cooked breakfast
For a special weekend treat, grill 1 lean sausage, 1 rasher of bacon, 1 large flat mushroom and 1 tomato, cut in half. Serve with 1 poached egg and 1 slice of wholemeal toast spread with Flora Light.

cals 517 | fat 25g | sat fat 12.3g | protein 21.7g

■ Shredded Wheat
A healthy cereal without any calorific nuts, honey or sugar coating! Simply serve 45g in a bowl with 125ml of semi-skimmed milk.

cals 210 | fat 3g | sat fat 1.5g | protein 9.5g

■ Boiled egg and soldiers
Boil an egg to your liking (3 minutes for very soft boiled, 8 for hard-boiled) and serve with 1 slice of wholemeal toast with Flora Light spread, cut into fingers.

cals 220 | fat 8.6g | sat fat 2.3g | protein 11.1g

■ Toast and jam
1 slice of wholemeal toast with a thin topping of Flora Light and some reduced-sugar jam.

cals 118 | fat 2.3g | sat fat 1.3g | protein 4.6g

■ Baked beans on toast
Sugar-free baked beans are a great source of fibre and protein. Have 1 small can on 1 slice of wholemeal toast.

cals 210 | fat 1.3g | sat fat 0.8g | protein 12.2g

138

LUNCH

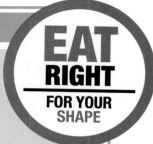

Crudités, houmous and pitta bread

Serve a small tub of low-fat houmous with a small warmed wholemeal pitta bread, cut into fingers. Add a few crudités such as some raw carrot sticks, raw cauliflower florets and a red pepper cut into strips.

cals 295 | fat 12g | sat fat 0g | protein 5.3g

Leek and potato soup

Buy a good leek and potato soup (check food label for fat content), or ideally make your own (see recipe on page 140). Serve with a wholemeal roll.

cals 176 | fat 10g | sat fat 5g | protein 7g

Chicken salad tortilla wrap

Warm 1 wholemeal tortilla wrap and fill with 3-4 slices cooked chicken, 1 handful of shredded lettuce, 1 chopped tomato and 1tbsp of low-fat mayonnaise.

cals 242 | fat 3.1g | sat fat 1.7g | protein 0g

Jacket potato with cottage cheese and chives

Bake or microwave a small jacket potato and top with 2-3tbsps of cottage cheese and chives.

cals 290 | fat 2.2g | sat fat 1g | protein 10g

Ham, cheese and salad roll

Choose a normal-size wholemeal roll (rather than a huge bap) and fill with 1 slice of lean ham, 2 slices of Cheddar cheese and a few lettuce leaves. Spread the top half of the roll with low-fat mayonnaise.

cals 295 | fat 6g | sat fat 2g | protein 14g

Prawn, cucumber and mayo sandwich

Take 2 pieces of thinly sliced wholemeal bread. Spread the bread with a thin layer of low-fat mayonnaise and fill with 80g of cooked, peeled prawns and 6 chunky slices of cucumber.

cals 279 | fat 5.6g | sat fat 2.5g | protein 23g

Herb omelette and green salad

Make an omelette with 2 eggs and 1tsp of Flora Light in an omelette pan. While cooking, sprinkle with 1tbsp each of chopped parsley and dill. Season and serve with a green salad.

cals 296 | fat 21g | sat fat 6g | protein 22g

Sardines and tomatoes on toast

Slice 1 large tomato and fry gently in a little olive oil. When softened, add 3 sardine fillets from a tin to warm through. Place the cooked tomatoes and the hot sardines on 1 slice of wholemeal toast spread with Flora Light.

cals 257 | fat 8.6g | sat fat 3.3g | protein 21.2g

Omelette

Whisk 2 eggs in a bowl, heat 1 small tbsp of Flora Light in an omelette pan and heat gently. Pour in the egg mixture and let the heat set the egg. Meanwhile, top the egg mixture with 1 thinly sliced mushroom, 1 thinly sliced tomato and 1tbsp of chopped crispy bacon and then fold in half. Finish off the cooking by putting the pan under a hot grill until golden.

cals 399 | fat 33g | sat fat 17g | protein 29g

Warm pitta bread filled with spicy chicken and salad

Fill one warmed pitta bread with 3-4 slices of hot tandoori chicken strips (available ready-cooked from supermarkets), 1 thinly sliced tomato, some shredded lettuce and 1tbsp of low-fat mayonnaise.

cals 276 | fat 9g | sat fat 3g | protein 22g

Grilled gammon steak and poached eggs

Grill a lean gammon steak for 3-4 minutes on each side and serve with 2 poached eggs.

cals 387 | fat 24.8g | sat fat 6.5g | protein 37.5g

Bagel with scrambled egg

Split a bagel (toasted if preferred) in half and top with 1 scrambled egg.

cals 283 | fat 8.5g | sat fat 3.9g | protein 14g

Salmon and egg salad

Make a mixed salad with chopped lettuce, 6 cherry tomatoes, cut in half, a few slices of cucumber and 6 olives. Place on plate and drizzle with a little olive oil. Decorate salad with 1 hard-boiled egg, cut into quarters, and top with a small tin of flaked red salmon.

cals 247 | fat 8.9g | sat fat 2g | protein 36g

Cream cheese, Ryvita crackers, celery and cherry tomatoes

Spread 2 Ryvitas with a small pot of low-fat cream cheese. Serve with 2-3 sticks of celery and cherry tomatoes drizzled with olive oil.

cals 118 | fat 2.8g | sat fat 1g | protein 10.2g

139

HOURGLASS

DINNER

■ Pork burgers with lemon and mint (serves 4)

Ingredients
- 450g minced lean pork
- ½ small onion, grated
- Zest and juice of 1 lemon
- 1 garlic clove, finely chopped
- 3tbsps mint, chopped
- Pinch of dried chilli flakes
- 1 egg white, beaten

Method
In a bowl, combine all the ingredients and mix thoroughly. Shape the mixture into 8 burgers about 2cm thick. Cover and leave in fridge for at least 1 hour to firm up. Heat a griddle or frying pan and cook for 4-5 minutes on each side. Serve with a mixed salad and low-fat mayonnaise.

cals 195 | fat 3.2g | sat fat 1g | protein 29.8g

■ Leek, potato and bacon soup (serves 4)

Ingredients
- 25g butter
- 7 rashers of streaky bacon, 3 chopped, 4 whole
- 1 onion, chopped
- 400g leeks, rinsed and chopped
- 3 small potatoes, peeled and diced
- 1L vegetable stock
- 142ml semi-skimmed milk

Method
Melt the butter in a large pan then fry the chopped bacon and onion on a medium heat, stirring occasionally, until golden. Add the leeks and potatoes, cover and turn down the heat. Cook gently for 5 minutes, shaking the pan occasionally to make sure it doesn't burn. Pour in the stock and bring to the boil. Cover and simmer for 20 minutes until the vegetables are soft. Meanwhile, grill the remaining bacon until crisp and crumble when cool enough to handle. Leave the soup to cool for a few minutes, then blend until smooth. Return to the pan, pour in the milk and stir well. Season to taste and serve with crisp bacon bits on top.

cals 176 | fat 10g | sat fat 5g | protein 7g

■ Quick Thai prawn curry (serves 4)

Ingredients
- 400ml reduced-fat coconut milk
- 200ml chicken stock
- 2tbsps Thai green curry paste
- 16 raw tiger prawns
- 6 spring onions, sliced diagonally
- 125g peas
- 2tbsps lime juice
- 8 cherry tomatoes
- 4tbsps fresh coriander, chopped
- 300g Basmati rice, cooked

Method
Stir together the coconut milk, stock and Thai curry paste in a wok or large frying pan and bring to the boil. Stir in the prawns, sliced spring onions, peas, lime juice and tomatoes and simmer it all for a further 4-5 minutes, until the prawns are pink and cooked. Finally, stir in the chopped coriander and season to taste. Serve with steamed or boiled rice.

cals 323 | fat 10.5g | sat fat 1g | protein 35g

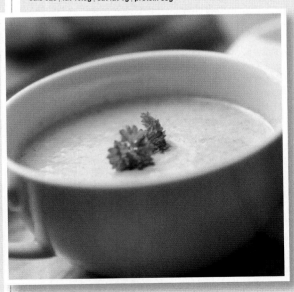

DINNER

EAT RIGHT
FOR YOUR **SHAPE**

■ Creamy vegetable risotto (serves 4)

Ingredients

- 1L vegetable stock
- 100g broccoli florets
- 100g asparagus, cut in half
- 500g broad beans
- 200g peas
- 2tbsps olive oil
- 1 onion, chopped
- 300g risotto rice
- 1tbsp pesto
- 25g pine nuts, toasted

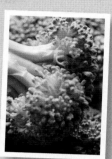

Method

Bring the vegetable stock to the boil in a large saucepan, then reduce the heat. Add the broccoli, asparagus, broad beans and peas, in that order, and simmer for 4-5 minutes until tender. Remove with a slotted spoon and set aside. Keep the stock simmering. Heat the oil in a large frying pan and add the chopped onion, fry for 2 minutes, then stir in the rice. Add 2-3 tablespoons of the hot stock and cook gently, stirring until the liquid is absorbed. Continue adding the stock spoon by spoon in this way until the mixture has a 'soupy' texture and the rice is tender. This will take about 20 minutes. Stir in the pesto and season to taste. Gently stir in the veg and heat through. Serve with toasted pine nuts scattered over the top.

cals 524 | fat 16g | sat fat 2g | protein 20g

■ Pork and chorizo casserole (serves 4)

Ingredients

- 2tbsps olive oil
- 2 onions, chopped
- 2 garlic cloves, crushed
- 1tbsp fresh rosemary
- 40g chorizo sausage, skinned and diced
- 2 red peppers, deseeded and chopped
- 40g sun-dried tomatoes, chopped
- 400g tin of chopped tomatoes
- 3tbsps white wine
- 1 pork tenderloin, cut into cubes
- 50g black or green olives, stoned

Method

Heat the oil in a casserole dish, add the onions, garlic and rosemary, and cook gently for about 15 minutes until soft and golden. Add the chorizo sausage and

red peppers and cook over a moderate heat for a couple of minutes. Add the sun-dried tomatoes and tinned tomatoes in their juice, and then the wine. Season with freshly ground black pepper, stir well and bring to a simmer. Add the pork and stir to coat with the sauce. Bring to the boil, then reduce the heat to a simmer. Cover and cook for 45 minutes until the pork is tender. Just before serving, stir in the olives and heat through.

cals 297 | fat 12g | sat fat 2.3g | protein 34g

■ Chicken with pesto, tomatoes and crème fraîche (serves 4)

Ingredients

- 1tbsp olive oil
- 4 boneless skinless chicken breasts
- 200g pack cherry tomatoes, halved
- 3tbsps pesto
- 3tbsps half-fat crème fraîche
- Fresh flat-leaf parsley, chopped

Method

Heat the oil in a non-stick frying pan. Add the chicken and fry on one side until golden. Turn it over and cook the other side. Continue cooking for 12-15 minutes until cooked completely through, then season. Add the tomatoes, and cook for a couple of minutes until they start to soften. Reduce the heat and stir in the pesto and crème fraîche to make a sauce. Scatter with a few pieces of chopped flat-leaf parsley, and serve with a green vegetable of your choice.

cals 263 | fat 13g | sat fat 6g | protein 36g

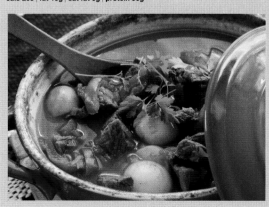

141

HOURGLASS

DINNER

■ Chicken and sweet potato curry (serves 2)
Ingredients
- 1tbsp olive oil
- 2tsps mild curry paste
- 2 skinless chicken breasts, cut into bite-size pieces
- 2 medium-sized sweet potatoes, peeled and cut into bite-size pieces
- 4tbsps split red lentils
- 300ml chicken stock
- 400ml can low-fat coconut milk
- 175g frozen peas
- 200g Basmati rice

Method
Heat the oil in a wok, stir in the curry paste and fry for 1 minute. Add the chicken, potatoes and lentils and stir to coat in the paste, then pour in the stock and coconut milk. Bring to the boil and simmer for 15 minutes. Add the peas, bring back to the boil and simmer for a further 4-5 minutes. Season to taste and serve with the rice.

cals 292 | fat 15g | sat fat 11g | protein 20g

■ Beef in ginger and garlic (serves 2)
Ingredients
- 2 pak choi, quartered
- 50g mangetout
- 1tsp sesame oil
- 1tbsp sunflower oil
- 1 large sirloin steak, trimmed of all fat and thinly sliced
- 1 inch root ginger, finely grated
- 1 garlic clove, crushed
- 4 spring onions, sliced
- 1tbsp soy sauce

Method
Steam the vegetables until tender, then toss with sesame oil and keep warm. Heat the sunflower oil in a wok, add the beef and brown. Add the ginger, crushed garlic and spring onions and cook for 2 minutes, stirring, then add the soy sauce and the vegetables.

cals 262 | fat 13g | sat fat 3.4g | protein 33.2g

■ Tasty fish stew (serves 4)
Ingredients
- 2tbsps olive oil
- 2 garlic cloves, crushed
- 1 small fennel bulb, shredded
- 1 pinch dried chilli flakes
- 1tsp paprika
- 150ml white wine
- 400g tin plum tomatoes, mashed
- 300ml chicken stock
- 400g skinless cod or haddock fillets, cut into chunks
- 250g cooked peeled prawns
- 1 bunch flat-leaf parsley, chopped

Method
Heat the olive oil in a large pan. Add the garlic and cook for 2 minutes, stirring, then add the fennel and cook for about 5 minutes until softened. Add the chilli and paprika, then pour in the wine and simmer until reduced. Add the tomatoes and stock, then simmer for 15-20 minutes until slightly thickened. Turn down the heat to a gentle simmer and add the white fish. Cover and cook for 3 minutes. Add the prawns for a couple of minutes until warm, and stir through the parsley.

cals 240 | fat 7.8g | sat fat 1.2g | protein 33g

■ Courgette and red onion frittata (Serves 3)
Ingredients
- 1 small red onion, halved and sliced
- 2 medium courgettes, sliced
- 2tbsps olive oil
- 6 eggs
- 50g mature Cheddar, grated

Method
Fry the onion and courgettes gently in a little olive oil for 10 minutes until soft and coloured. Beat the eggs, then mix in the cheese and veg. Heat some oil in a small non-stick frying pan and pour in the egg mix. Stir once, then leave to cook until the base is firm and it's nearly set. Slide under a hot grill until puffed and golden. Cut into wedges and serve with a green salad.

cals 489 | fat 38.9g | sat fat 12g | protein 30g

142

DINNER

▪ Spicy lamb koftas (serves 8)
Ingredients
- 2tbsps olive oil
- 1 onion, chopped
- 1tbsp fresh ginger, grated
- 2 garlic cloves, crushed
- 1tsp ground mixed peppercorns
- 1 level tsp ground cumin
- 1tsp chilli powder
- 500g lamb mince
- 1 egg, beaten

Method
Heat 1 tablespoon of oil in a large frying pan, fry the onions with the ginger, garlic and spices for 5 minutes until soft, then put into a large bowl to cool. Mix together the lamb and egg with the onion mix and season. Shape the mixture into 12 patties. Heat the remaining oil in the pan and fry for 4 minutes each side, or until cooked through. Serve with a green salad.

cals 115 | fat 4g | sat fat 2.8g | protein 10g

▪ Roasted duck legs with sweet potato (serves 6)
Ingredients
- 6 duck legs, pricked all over with a fork
- 12 shallots
- 2 bay leaves
- ¼tsp allspice
- 300ml white wine
- 2 large sweet potatoes, cubed
- Knob of butter
- 1 small bunch parsley, chopped

Method
Heat the oven to 190°C/370°F/ Gas Mark 5. Put the duck legs in a single layer in a large roasting tin and tuck the shallots and bay leaves around them. Mix the allspice with ½ teaspoon of salt and sprinkle a little on each leg. Roast for 1 hour. Spoon off almost all the fat, then add the wine and return to the oven for 20 minutes to finish cooking. Meanwhile, boil the sweet potatoes until tender, then mash with a small knob of butter and season well. Put a scoop of mash on each plate and lean a duck leg up against it, spoon some shallots and sauce around them and sprinkle with parsley.

cals 388 | fat 15.2g | sat fat 6.1g | protein 29g

▪ Baked salmon with a Parmesan crust (serves 4)
Ingredients
- 4 salmon fillets
- Butter, to grease
- 50g fresh wholemeal breadcrumbs
- 2tbsps chopped parsley
- Juice of ½ a lime
- 1tbsp olive oil
- 40g Parmesan cheese

Method
Heat the oven to 180°C/350°F/Gas Mark 4. Season and put the salmon fillets on a lightly buttered non-stick baking tray. Whizz the breadcrumbs, parsley, lime juice, olive oil and Parmesan in a food processor. Cover the salmon with the breadcrumbs and bake in the oven for 10-12 minutes until the salmon is cooked through and the breadcrumbs golden. Serve with a salad.

cals 338 | fat 19.5g | sat fat 5.9g | protein 31.5g

▪ Roasted tomatoes and goat's cheese (serves 2)
Ingredients
- 250g bag spinach
- A pinch of freshly grated nutmeg
- 4 slices prosciutto
- 3 large tomatoes, halved
- 1 heaped tbsp crème fraîche
- 50g goat's cheese, chopped

Method
Heat oven to 180°C/350°F/Gas Mark 4. Put the spinach leaves in a hot pan, season well, then cover and leave to wilt for 1 minute, stirring once or twice. Put the spinach in the bottom of a gratin dish then sprinkle with nutmeg. Drape the prosciutto slices over and around the spinach, then sit the tomato halves on top, cut-side up. Dot the crème fraîche over the whole dish, scatter with the goat's cheese, and then season with more pepper. Bake for 10-15 minutes until the cheese is melting into the crème fraîche and the edges are starting to bubble. Scoop out of the dish and serve with a green salad.

cals 239 | fat 18g | sat fat 9.2g | protein 15g

143

BOY

Boy shapes often crave savoury, salty snacks, junk foods and high-GI carbs, such as pasta and white bread. To make your diet healthier, you should choose lean meats, poultry, fish and shellfish, and complex carbs like fresh fruit, veg and wholemeal bread instead. It's also important to include foods that are good sources of omega-3, like salmon, halibut, sardines, avocados, nuts and olive oil.

BREAKFAST

■ Natural yoghurt, fruit and toasted almonds
Cut up 3 of your favourite fruits and mix with 3tbsps of natural yoghurt. Sprinkle with toasted almonds.
cals 231 | fat 2.5g | sat fat 0.5g | protein 12g

■ Scrambled eggs and bacon on toast
Grill 1 rasher of back bacon. Scramble 2 eggs with a dash of skimmed milk. Serve on 1 slice of wholemeal toast with the bacon.
cals 295 | fat 19.3g | sat fat 5.5g | protein 29g

■ Cereal with fruit
Mix 40g of bran flakes or All Bran with 2-3 chopped prunes or dried apricots. Serve with 125ml of semi-skimmed milk.
cals 298 | fat 2.9g | sat fat 0.8g | protein 9.5g

■ Porridge with yoghurt and honey
Make a bowl of porridge in the microwave or on the hob with 40g of oats (not powder) and semi-skimmed milk, according to packet instructions. Serve with 1tbsp of natural yoghurt in the middle, and a drizzle of honey.
cals 284 | fat 5.9g | sat fat 1.8g | protein 7.7g

■ Button mushrooms on toast
Pan-fry 45-50g of button mushrooms in 1tsp of butter and 1tsp of olive oil. Serve on 1 slice of wholemeal toast with Flora Light spread.
cals 189 | fat 14g | sat fat 3.2g | protein 12.8g

■ Muesli with extra nuts
A bowl of sugar-free muesli (50g) served with 1tbsp each of toasted almonds and walnuts, and 125ml of semi-skimmed milk.
cals 362 | fat 6.2g | sat fat 1.8g | protein 13g

■ Warm bagel and scrambled eggs
Scramble 2 eggs with 1tsp of butter and serve on a toasted bagel.
cals 298 | fat 9.6g | sat fat 2g | protein 12.3g

■ Wholemeal muffin
Toast 1 wholemeal muffin, cut in half and top with Flora Light spread.
cals 145 | fat 3.5g | sat fat 1g | protein 8g

■ Breakfast fruit and veg smoothie
Blend 1 chopped apple, 4 carrots, 2 sticks of celery and 2 kiwis into a smoothie.
cals 145 | fat 0g | sat fat 0g | protein 4g

■ Cooked breakfast
For a special weekend treat, grill 1 lean sausage, 1 rasher of bacon, 1 large flat mushroom and 1 tomato cut into 2 halves. Serve with 1 poached egg and a slice of wholemeal toast spread with Flora Light.
cals 517 | fat 25g | sat fat 12.3g | protein 21.7g

■ Weetabix
A healthy cereal without any calorific nuts, honey or sugar coating! Simply serve 2 Weetabix biscuits in a bowl with 125ml of semi-skimmed milk.
cals 195 | fat 3g | sat fat 1.5g | protein 9g

■ Boiled egg and soldiers
Cook 1 egg to your liking (somewhere between 3 minutes for very soft-boiled and 8 minutes for completely hard-boiled) with 1 slice of wholemeal toast and Flora Light spread.
cals 220 | fat 8.6g | sat fat 2.3g | protein 11.1g

■ Toast and marmalade
Spread 1 slice wholemeal toast with low-sugar marmalade and Flora Light.
cals 132 | fat 1.3g | sat fat 0.8g | protein 4.6g

■ Baked beans on toast
Baked beans are a great source of fibre and protein. Choose the low-sugar option (1 small can), heat through and serve on 1 slice of wholemeal toast.
cals 210 | fat 1.3g | sat fat 0.8g | protein 12.2g

144

LUNCH

Crudités, low-fat olive houmous and pitta bread
Serve 25g of olive houmous with 1 warmed wholemeal pitta bread cut into fingers. Add a few crudités, such as some raw carrot sticks, raw cauliflower florets and a red pepper, cut into strips.
cals 198 | fat 4g | sat fat 2g | protein 9g

Tomato soup
Buy a good tomato soup (check fat content), or make your own (see page 147). Serve with a wholemeal roll.
cals 213 | fat 14g | sat fat 7g | protein 8g

Chicken salad tortilla wrap
Warm 1 wholemeal tortilla wrap and fill with 3-4 slices of cooked chicken, a handful of shredded lettuce, 1 chopped tomato and 1tbsp of low-fat mayonnaise.
cals 242 | fat 3.1g | sat fat 1.7g | protein 0g

Jacket potato with tuna mayo
Bake or microwave a small potato and top with 1 small tin of tuna (in water) mixed with 2tbsps of low-fat mayo.
cals 298 | fat 1.8g | sat fat 0.9g | protein 9.5g

Cheese, cucumber and onion roll
Fill a normal-sized wholemeal roll with 2tbsps of grated cheese, some chopped cucumber and ½ a small chopped onion. Top with low-fat mayo.
cals 296 | fat 7g | sat fat 2.5g | protein 19.8g

Egg and mayo sandwich
Fill 2 pieces of thinly sliced wholemeal bread with 1 chopped hard-boiled egg mixed with low-fat mayo.
cals 282 | fat 4.8g | sat fat 2g | protein 23g

Cheese and mushroom omelette with green salad
Pan-fry 6 sliced mushrooms in an omelette pan with 1tsp of Flora Light. Then add 2 beaten eggs and make an omelette, sprinkling over 1tbsp of grated cheese while cooking. Serve with a green salad.
cals 296 | fat 25g | sat fat 10.2g | protein 28g

Sardines and tomatoes on toast
Slice 1 large tomato and pan-fry gently in a little olive oil. When softened, add 3 sardine fillets from a tin to warm through. Place the cooked tomatoes and the hot sardines on 1 slice of wholemeal toast.
cals 257 | fat 8.6g | sat fat 3.3g | protein 21.2g

Omelette
Whisk 2 eggs in a bowl, heat 1 small tbsp of Flora Light in an omelette pan and heat gently. Pour in the egg mixture and let the heat set the egg. Meanwhile, top with strips of ham (cut from 1 slice), 1 thinly sliced tomato and 1tbsp of grated Cheddar cheese. Finish off the cooking under a hot grill, with the omelette still in the pan, until golden on top.
cals 378 | fat 32g | sat fat 12g | protein 27g

Warm pitta with spicy chicken strips and salad
Fill 1 warmed wholemeal pitta bread with 3 hot tandoori chicken strips (available at supermarkets), 1 thinly sliced tomato, some shredded lettuce and 1tbsp of low-fat mayonnaise.
cals 298 | fat 10.2g | sat fat 4g | protein 23g

Waldorf salad
Cut 1 apple and 2 sticks of celery into chunks. Mix with 2tbsps of low-fat mayonnaise and 6-8 toasted walnut halves. Serve on fresh salad leaves.
cals | 120 | fat 7g | sat fat 1g | protein 15g

Hoisin chicken tortilla wrap
Mix 200g cooked chicken strips with 1tbsp of hoisin sauce, making sure that they're all well coated, then spread out on an ovenproof dish and grill until sizzling. Warm 1 tortilla wrap according to packet instructions. Spread the tortilla with another tablespoon of hoisin sauce, then wrap up the chicken with some chopped cucumber and 2 chopped spring onions. Cut in half and enjoy while still warm.
cals 302 | fat 6g | sat fat 2g | protein 33g

Egg and bacon salad
Make a mixed salad with chopped lettuce, 6 cherry tomatoes, cut in half, and a few slices of cucumber. Then chop 1 hard-boiled egg and 2 rashers of back bacon, cooked to your liking, and pop on the salad.
cals 265 | fat 13g | sat fat 6g | protein 32g

Cream cheese, Ryvita crackers, celery and baby pickled onions
Serve 2 Ryvita or other low-fat crispbreads with 1 small pot of low-fat cream cheese, half a dozen baby pickled onions and 2-3 sticks of chopped celery for a Scandinavian-style lunch.
cals 119 | fat 1.7g | sat fat 0.8g | protein 13g

145

BOY

DINNER

■ Little meatballs with couscous (serves 4)
Ingredients
- 500g lean minced beef
- 1 red onion, chopped
- 2 garlic cloves, crushed
- 2tsps ground cumin
- 1tsp ground cinnamon
- 1tbsp olive oil
- 2 x 400g tins chopped tomatoes
- 200ml beef stock
- ½ bunch of parsley, chopped
- 200g Basmati rice

Method
Put the beef, onion, garlic and spices in a bowl and season. Mix well and form into little meatballs (approximately 30). Heat the olive oil in a large pan and add the meatballs in batches, frying until they're browned all over. Set aside, add the tomatoes and stock to the pan, then season. Simmer for 10 minutes, then return the meatballs and cook for another 20 minutes until the sauce has thickened. Stir in the parsley, and serve with rice.

cals 432 | fat 24g | sat fat 9g | protein 28g

■ Thai prawn salad (serves 2)
Ingredients
- 180g lettuce leaves, shredded
- 80g cucumber, diced
- 1 carrot, peeled and grated
- 60g bean sprouts
- 2tbsps olive oil
- 1 clove of garlic, crushed
- 1 stick of lemongrass, inner stalk chopped
- Small bunch coriander, chopped
- 200g raw prawns, peeled
- 1 lime
- 1dsp sweet chilli sauce

Method
Arrange the lettuce, cucumber, carrots and bean sprouts on individual plates. Heat 1 tablespoon of olive oil in a wok and gently cook the garlic and lemongrass

for about 30 seconds. Add the prawns and fry over a high heat for 1-2 minutes, stirring constantly. Remove from the pan and divide between the salad vegetables. Squeeze 2 tablespoons of lime juice into the pan and add the coriander, the remaining olive oil and the chilli sauce. Stir for 1 minute then pour over the salad.

cals 282 | fat 7g | sat fat 2g | protein 18g

■ Haddock and spinach with a creamy sauce (serves 2)
Ingredients
- 1tsp sunflower or vegetable oil
- 2 haddock fillets
- 250g bag spinach
- 2tbsps reduced-fat crème fraîche
- Juice of ½ a lemon
- 1tsp capers, drained
- 2tbsps flat-leaf parsley, chopped

Method
Heat the oil in a pan, season the haddock, then fry for 4 minutes each side until golden and the flesh flakes easily. Leave to rest on a plate while you cook the spinach. Put the leaves into the hot pan, season then cover and leave to wilt for 1 minute, stirring once. Spoon the spinach on to plates and top with the haddock. Gently heat the crème fraîche in the pan with a squeeze of the lemon juice, capers and parsley, then season. Spoon the sauce over the fish and serve.

cals 321 | fat 20g | sat fat 5g | protein 32g

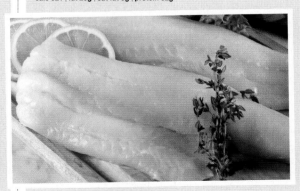

146

DINNER

■ Hearty tomato soup (serves 4)

Ingredients
- 1tbsp olive oil
- 2 garlic cloves, crushed
- 5 soft, sun-dried tomatoes in oil, roughly chopped
- 3 x 400g cans plum tomatoes
- 500ml chicken or vegetable stock
- 142ml pot sour cream

Method
Heat the oil in a large pan, then add the garlic and soften for a few minutes over a low heat. Add the sun-dried tomatoes, tinned tomatoes and stock and bring to a simmer. Let the soup bubble gently for 10 minutes until the tomatoes have broken down a little. Whizz with a hand blender, adding half the pot of sour cream as you go. Taste and season if necessary. Serve in bowls with a little more sour cream.

cals 213 | fat 14g | sat fat 7g | protein 8g

■ Chicken and red pepper stir-fry (serves 2)

Ingredients
- 3tbsps groundnut or sunflower oil
- 2 garlic cloves, thinly sliced
- 1 small red pepper, deseeded and thinly sliced
- 2 chicken breasts, cut into strips
- 2tbsps soy sauce
- 100g bag baby spinach leaves

Method
Heat a wok, add 2 tablespoons of oil and the garlic. Stir-fry until the pieces just turn golden, then spoon on to kitchen paper to drain. Add the pepper and stir-fry for 1 minute until slightly softened, then spoon out and set aside. Add the remaining tablespoon of oil. Heat, then add the chicken and stir-fry for 5 minutes, or until cooked. Add the soy sauce. Pop in the spinach and stir-fry until it begins to wilt. Return the peppers and garlic to the wok and serve.

cals 270 | fat 18g | sat fat 3g | protein 25g

■ Spanish omelette (serves 8)

Ingredients
- 400g bag spinach leaves
- 3tbsps olive oil
- 1 large onion, finely sliced
- 2 potatoes, peeled and finely sliced
- 10 eggs

Method
Heat the grill to high. Put the spinach leaves into a hot pan, season, then cover and leave to wilt for 1 minute, stirring once or twice. Heat the oil in a non-stick frying pan and cook the onion and potato for about 10 minutes until the potato is soft. Beat the eggs together in a large bowl and season. Stir the spinach into the potatoes, then pour in the eggs and leave to cook until set most of the way through. Put the omelette under the grill to crisp the top, and cook until golden. Cut into wedges and serve.

cals 209 | fat 13g | sat fat 3g | protein 12g

■ Fresh tuna steak with roasted tomatoes (serves 2)

Ingredients
- 2tbsps olive oil
- 4tbsps balsamic vinegar
- 250g cherry tomatoes on the vine
- 2 tuna steaks (around 150g each)
- Salad leaves

Method
Heat the oven to 180°C/350°F/Gas Mark 4. Mix the olive oil with the balsamic vinegar and season. Put the tomatoes in a roasting tin and pour most, but not all, of the balsamic mixture over the top. Roast for 15 minutes. Meanwhile, heat a griddle pan. Season and lightly oil the tuna steaks, then cook for 2 minutes each side. Serve with the tomatoes, salad and the rest of the balsamic oil drizzled over the top.

cals 350 | fat 18.6g | sat fat 3.1g | protein 37g

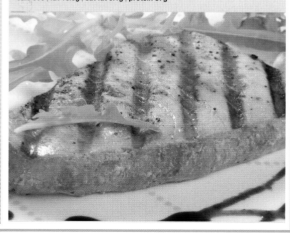

147

BOY

DINNER

■ **Couscous salad (serves 2)**
Ingredients
• 100g couscous
• 200ml hot vegetable stock
• 2 spring onions
• 1 red pepper
• ½ a cucumber
• 2tbsps pesto
• 50g Feta cheese, cubed
• 2tbsps toasted pine nuts

Method
Put the couscous into a large bowl, pour over the stock and cover. Leave for 10 minutes, until it is fluffy and all the stock has been absorbed. Meanwhile, thinly slice the onions and pepper and dice the cucumber. Add these to the cooked couscous, fork through the pesto, crumble in the Feta, and sprinkle over the pine nuts.

cals 327 | fat 17g | sat fat 5g | protein 13g

■ **Spicy rice (serves 4)**
Ingredients
• 1tbsp olive oil
• 2 garlic cloves, crushed
• 2tbsps medium curry paste
• 250g Basmati rice
• 450ml vegetable stock
• 400g can chickpeas, drained and rinsed
• A handful of raisins
• 175g frozen leaf spinach, thawed
• A handful of cashew nuts
• ½ a cup of natural yoghurt, to serve

Method
Heat the oil in a large, non-stick pan, then fry the garlic and curry paste over a medium heat for 1 minute. Put the rice in the pan with the stock, chickpeas and raisins and stir with a fork to stop the rice from clumping, being careful not to scratch your pan in the process. Season, then cover and bring to the boil. Reduce to a medium heat and cook for 12-15 minutes or until all the liquid has been absorbed. Squeeze any excess water from the spinach with your hands, and add to the pan along with 2 tablespoons of hot water. Fluff up the rice with a

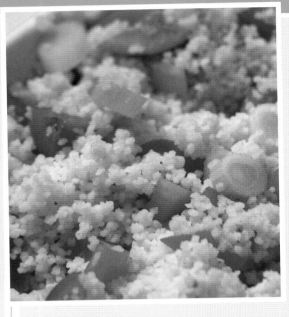

fork, making sure the spinach is mixed in well. Toss in the cashews. Serve, drizzled with natural yoghurt.

cals 378 | fat 9.2g | sat fat 1g | protein 13g

■ **Haddock fillets with tomatoes and black olives (serves 4)**
Ingredients
• 75g black olives in oil, stones removed
• 1 large onion, roughly chopped
• 400g can chopped tomatoes
• 4 boneless haddock fillets
• 1tbsp fresh flat-leaf parsley, chopped

Method
Preheat the oven to 180°C /350°F/Gas Mark 4. Heat 1 tablespoon of the oil from the olives in an ovenproof pan. Add the onion and stir, leave to cook for 2 minutes and stir again. Add the tomatoes and season. Bring to the boil, then add the olives. Place the fish, on the sauce and drizzle over a splash more oil. Bake in the oven for 15 minutes. Sprinkle with parsley and serve.

cals 223 | fat 6g | sat fat 1g | protein 34g

148

DINNER

■ Lemon chicken (serves 4)

Ingredients
- 4 chicken breast fillets
- 1 large lemon
- 2tsps fresh thyme leaves
- 1½tbsps clear honey
- 200g Basmati rice

Method
Preheat the grill to high and lightly oil a shallow, heatproof dish. Put the chicken in the dish and season. Grill for 5 minutes. While the chicken is cooking, cut 4 thin slices of lemon. Turn the chicken fillets over and put a slice of lemon on top of each one. Sprinkle over the thyme and a little more seasoning, then drizzle with the honey. Mix the juice from the remaining lemon with 2 tablespoons of water and pour over. Return to the grill for 10 minutes until the chicken is golden and cooked through. Serve the chicken and the sticky juices with Basmati rice and a green vegetable of your choice.

cals 195 | fat 5g | sat fat 1g | protein 34g

■ Healthy tuna burgers (serves 2)

Ingredients
- 200g fresh tuna steaks
- 1 garlic clove, finely chopped
- 1 small piece fresh ginger, peeled and finely chopped
- 1tbsp soy sauce
- A handful of coriander leaves, chopped
- 1tbsp olive oil
- To serve: burger buns, lettuce leaves, sliced tomato and ripe avocado

Method
Chop the tuna until it is roughly minced and put into a bowl with the garlic, ginger, soy sauce and coriander. Mix well, then shape into two burgers. Place these on a plate and put in the freezer for 10 minutes to firm up. Heat the oil in a non-stick frying pan, cook the burgers for 1-2 minutes on each side. Serve in toasted buns with suggestions above (will increase calorie count).

cals 137 | fat 5g | sat fat 1g | protein 13g

■ Mini chicken kebabs and avocado salsa (serves 2)

Ingredients
- 2 skinless chicken breasts, cubed
- 2tsps sesame seeds
- 1 lemon (zest and juice)
- 1 avocado
- ½ a cucumber
- 1 chilli, finely chopped
- A handful of coriander leaves
- 1tbsp olive oil

Method
Toss the chicken with the sesame seeds, lemon zest and some salt and pepper. Thread on to skewers. Chop the avocado and cucumber into cubes and toss with the lemon juice, chilli and coriander leaves. Drizzle on a little oil and season. Drizzle the rest of the oil over the chicken and grill until cooked through. Serve with the salsa.

cals 355 | fat 21g | sat fat 3g | protein 36g

■ Sausage and bean hotpot (serves 4)

Ingredients
- 8 lean sausages
- 2 x 420g cans mixed beans
- 2 x 400g cans chopped tomatoes
- 1tsp dried basil
- 2tsps dried oregano
- 1tbsp sugar

Method
Heat a large non-stick frying pan and brown the sausages for 3-5 minutes over a medium to high heat. Drain the beans, and add to the pan with the chopped tomatoes, herbs and sugar. Season well and bring to the boil. Simmer for 10 minutes until the sausages are cooked through and the sauce has thickened.

cals 352 | fat 16g | sat fat 4g | protein 21g

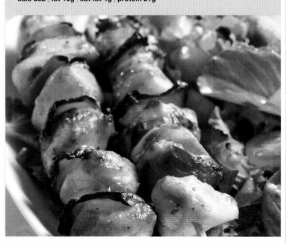

149

APPLE

Apple shapes tend to crave starchy, flour-based carbs, such as bread and biscuits, as well as fatty, spicy foods and salty snacks. You should opt instead for complex carbs, such as fresh fruit and veg (except potatoes) and proteins like beans and pulses, lean meat and poultry, wholewheat cereals, eggs, fish and shellfish. Choose low-fat dairy products and use olive oil for cooking and dressing food.

BREAKFAST

■ Natural yoghurt, fruit and toasted sunflower seeds
Cut up 3 of your favourite fruits (such as a banana, a satsuma and a few strawberries) and mix with 3tbsps of low-fat natural yoghurt. Sprinkle with some toasted sunflower seeds.
cals 229 | fat 2.5g | sat fat 0.5g | protein 11g

■ Scrambled eggs and ham
Scramble 2 eggs with a dash of skimmed milk and add seasoning to taste. Serve with 2 thin slices of good quality, lean ham.
cals 262 | fat 16.3g | sat fat 3.5g | protein 25g

■ Cereal with fruit
Mix together 40g of bran flakes or All Bran with 2-3 chopped dried apricots and 1tsp of chopped toasted almonds. Serve with 125ml of semi-skimmed milk.
cals 287 | fat 3.9g | sat fat 1.8g | protein 10.5g

■ Porridge and fruit yoghurt
Make a bowl of porridge in the microwave or on the hob with 40g of oats (not powder) and semi-skimmed milk, according to packet instructions. Serve with 1tbsp low-fat/low-sugar fruit yoghurt in the middle.
cals 270 | fat 5.5g | sat fat 1g | protein 6.7g

■ Grilled mushrooms and poached egg on toast
Grill 2 large Portobello mushrooms and serve on top of 1 slice of wholemeal toast with 1 poached egg.
cals 223 | fat 15.6g | sat fat 3.9g | protein 11.7g

■ Muesli with grated apple
A bowl of sugar-free muesli (50g) served with 1 peeled, grated apple and 125ml of semi-skimmed milk.
cals 350 | fat 5g | sat fat 1.5g | protein 10g

■ Smoked salmon and scrambled eggs
Scramble 2 eggs with 1tsp of butter over a gentle heat and serve with 25g of smoked salmon cut into thin strips, and chopped chives if desired.
cals 234 | fat 8.6g | sat fat 1.7g | protein 8.9g

■ Wholemeal muffin
Toast 1 wholemeal muffin, and top each half with Flora Light spread.
cals 145 | fat 3.5g | sat fat 1g | protein 8g

■ Breakfast fruit smoothie
Blend together 3 passion fruits (seeds only), 1 banana, 1 small mango (peeled, stoned and chopped) and 300ml of orange juice to make a smoothie.
cals 162 | fat 0g | sat fat 0g | protein 3g

■ Cooked breakfast
For a special weekend treat, grill 1 lean sausage, 1 rasher of bacon, 1 large flat mushroom and 1 tomato, cut in half. Serve with 1 poached egg and 1 slice of wholemeal toast spread with Flora Light.
cals 517 | fat 25g | sat fat 12.3g | protein 21.7g

■ Mini Shredded Wheat
A healthy cereal without any calorific nuts, honey or sugar coating! Simply serve 45g in a bowl with 125ml of semi-skimmed milk.
cals 210 | fat 3g | sat fat 1.5g | protein 9.5g

■ Boiled egg and soldiers
1 boiled egg and a 1 slice of wholemeal toast topped with Flora Light spread, cut into fingers.
cals 220 | fat 8.6g | sat fat 2.3g | protein 11.1g

■ Toast and Marmite
1 slice of wholemeal toast topped with a thin spread of Flora Light and Marmite.
cals 118 | fat 2.3g | sat fat 1.3g | protein 4.6g

■ Baked beans on toast
Baked beans are a great source of fibre and protein. Choose the low-fat/low-sugar option (1 small can) and serve on 1 slice of wholemeal toast.
cals 210 | fat 1.3g | sat fat 0.8g | protein 12.2g

150

LUNCH

■ Crudités and Philadelphia Light with chives and pitta bread

Serve 25g of Philadelphia Light with a small, warm wholemeal pitta bread cut into fingers. Add a few crudités, such as raw carrot sticks, raw cauliflower florets and a red pepper, cut into strips.

cals 195 | fat 4g | sat fat 2g | protein 8g

■ Vegetable soup

Buy a good vegetable soup (check the fat content on the label), or ideally make your own (see recipe on page 154). Serve with a wholemeal roll.

cals 374 | fat 9g | sat fat 4g | protein 12g

■ Chicken salad tortilla wrap

Warm 1 wholemeal tortilla wrap and fill with 3-4 slices cooked chicken, 1 handful of shredded lettuce, 1 chopped tomato and 1tbsp of low-fat mayonnaise.

cals 242 | fat 3.1g | sat fat 1.7g | protein 0g

■ Jacket potato with cottage cheese

Bake or microwave 1 small jacket potato and top with 2tbsps of cottage cheese.

cals 290 | fat 1.2g | sat fat 0.5g | protein 6.5g

■ Ham and salad roll

Choose 1 normal-size wholemeal roll (rather than a huge bap) and fill with lean ham and salad of your choice. Spread the top half of the roll with low-fat mayonnaise.

cals 275 | fat 5g | sat fat 1.5g | protein 13.3g

■ Salmon and cucumber sandwich

Make a sandwich from two pieces of thinly sliced wholemeal bread, 1 small tin of salmon and 6-8 slices of cucumber. Spread the bread with a thin layer of low-fat mayonnaise.

cals 282 | fat 4.8g | sat fat 2g | protein 23g

■ Ham omelette and green salad

Melt 1tsp of Flora Light in a pan and make an omelette with 2 eggs. Add 1 slice of ham cut into small chunks. Serve with a green salad.

cals 297 | fat 26g | sat fat 10.2g | protein 26g

■ Sardines and tomatoes on toast

Slice 1 large tomato and pan-fry gently in a little olive oil. When softened, add 3 sardine fillets from a tin to warm through. Place the cooked tomatoes and hot sardines on 1 slice of wholemeal toast spread with Flora Light.

cals 257 | fat 8.6g | sat fat 3.3g | protein 21.2g

■ Omelette

Whisk 2 eggs in a bowl, heat 1 small tablespoon of Flora Light in an omelette pan and heat gently. Pour in the egg mixture, stir briefly, and then let the heat set the egg. Top the egg mixture with 4 thin slices of chorizo, 1 thinly sliced tomato and 1tbsp of grated Cheddar cheese. Finish off the cooking under a hot grill, with the omelette still in the pan, until nicely golden on top.

cals 399 | fat 36g | sat fat 17g | protein 28g

■ Warmed pitta bread filled with chicken salad

Fill 1 warm pitta bread with 4 slices of lean cooked chicken, 1 thinly sliced tomato, some shredded lettuce and 1tbsp of low-fat mayonnaise.

cals 273 | fat 8.1g | sat fat 1.2g | protein 19g

■ Grilled gammon, poached egg and tomato

Grill a piece of lean gammon (cut off any excess fat!) for 3-4 minutes on each side and serve with 1 poached egg and a grilled tomato.

cals 289 | fat 20.3g | sat fat 4.2g | protein 31.5g

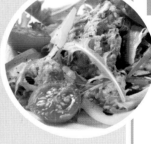

■ Warm bagel with scrambled egg

Split a bagel (toasted if preferred) in half and top with 1 scrambled egg.

cals 305 | fat 9g | sat fat 3.5g | protein 20g

■ Tuna salad

Make a mixed salad with chopped lettuce, 6 cherry tomatoes cut in half, a few slices of cucumber and 6 olives. Drizzle with a little olive oil. Top the salad with a small tin of flaked tuna (in water).

cals 175 | fat 4g | sat fat 1.2g | protein 25.3g

■ Cottage cheese with chives, Ryvita crackers, celery and apple

Top 2 Ryvitas with 1 small pot of cottage cheese with chives (or snip over your own) and serve with 2-3 sticks of celery and 1 sliced apple.

cals 110 | fat 1.8g | sat fat 0.9g | protein 9g

APPLE

DINNER

■ Little spicy meatballs with couscous (serves 4)
Ingredients
- 500g lean minced lamb
- 1 red onion, grated
- 2 garlic cloves, crushed
- 2cm piece root ginger, grated
- 1 pinch dried chilli flakes
- 2tsps ground cumin
- 1tsp ground cinnamon
- 1tbsp olive oil
- 2 x 400g tins plum tomatoes, mashed
- 200ml chicken stock
- 200g couscous

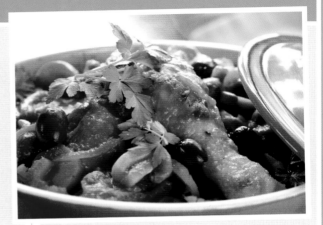

Method
Put the lamb, onion, half the garlic, half the ginger and half the spices in a bowl and season. Mix well and form into little meatballs (about 30). Heat the oil in a large non-stick pan and add the meatballs in batches, frying until browned all over. Spoon out, then add the rest of the garlic, ginger and spices and cook for 2 minutes. Add the tomatoes and stock and season. Simmer for 10 minutes, then return the meatballs and cook for another 20 minutes, until sauce is thickened. Serve with couscous made according to packet instructions.

cals 504 | fat 30g | sat fat 14g | protein 30g

■ Chicken and haricot bean casserole (serves 4)
Ingredients
- 2tbsps olive oil
- 400g skinless chicken thighs
- 1 onion, chopped
- 3 carrots, chopped
- 3 celery sticks, chopped
- ½tsp dried thyme
- 1 bay leaf
- 600ml chicken stock
- 2 x 400g cans haricot beans, drained
- 1tbsp fresh flat-leaf parsley, chopped

Method
Heat the oil in a large pan, add the chicken and fry until lightly browned. Add the veg, frying for a few minutes.

Stir in the herbs and stock. Bring to the boil. Stir well, reduce the heat, cover and cook for 40 minutes, until the chicken is tender. Stir the beans into the pan, and simmer for 5 minutes. Stir in the parsley, season to taste and serve with broccoli or peas.

cals 291 | fat 9g | sat fat 2g | protein 30g

■ Chicken, goat's cheese and tomato bake (serves 4)
Ingredients
- 4 skinless chicken breasts
- 150g firm goat's cheese
- 1 bunch of thyme
- 500g cherry tomatoes
- 1tbsp olive oil
- 1 splash of white wine
- 300g Basmati rice

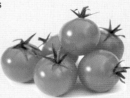

Method
Heat oven to 190°C/370°F/Gas Mark 5. Split each chicken breast slightly and stuff with a slice of the goat's cheese and a sprig of thyme. Put in a shallow ovenproof dish. Halve the cherry tomatoes and scatter them around the chicken with a few more sprigs of thyme, a drizzle of olive oil and splash of white wine. Season with freshly ground pepper. Bake for 25-30 minutes until the chicken is tender and golden. Serve with boiled Basmati rice.

cals 330 | fat 16g | sat fat 8g | protein 40g

DINNER

■ Salmon with a creamy spinach sauce (serves 2)

Ingredients
- 1tsp olive oil
- 2 skinless salmon fillets
- 250g spinach
- 2tbsps low-fat crème fraîche
- Juice of ½ a lemon
- 1tsp capers, drained
- 2tbsps flat-leaf parsley, chopped
- Lemon wedges, to serve

Method
Heat the oil in a pan, season the salmon on both sides, then fry for 4 minutes on each side until golden and flaky. Leave to rest on a plate while you cook the spinach. Tip the leaves into the hot pan, season well, then cover and leave to wilt for 1 minute, stirring once or twice. Spoon the spinach on to plates and top with the salmon. Gently heat the crème fraîche in the pan with a squeeze of lemon juice, capers and parsley, then season to taste. Be careful not to let it boil. Spoon the sauce over the fish and serve with lemon wedges.

cals 321 | fat 20g | sat fat 5g | protein 32g

■ Chicken casserole (serves 4)

Ingredients
- 2tbsps olive oil
- 2 onions, chopped
- 2 garlic cloves, crushed
- 1tbsp fresh rosemary
- 2 red peppers, deseeded and chopped
- 40g sun-dried tomatoes, chopped
- 400g tin chopped tomatoes
- 3tbsps white wine
- 4 skinless chicken breasts
- 50g stoned black olives

Method
Heat the oil in a casserole dish, add the onions, garlic and rosemary, and cook gently for about 15 minutes until soft and golden. Add the red peppers and cook over a moderate heat for a couple of minutes. Add the sun-dried tomatoes, tinned tomatoes and wine. Season with freshly ground black pepper, stir well and bring to a simmer. Add the chicken and stir to coat with the sauce. Bring to the boil then reduce to a simmer. Cover and cook for 30 minutes until the chicken is tender. Just before serving, stir in the olives and heat through.

cals 272 | fat 9g | sat fat 1.8g | protein 29g

■ Thai chicken salad (serves 4)

Ingredients
- 350g lettuce leaves, shredded
- 175g cucumber, diced
- 2 carrots, peeled and grated
- 115g bean sprouts
- 2tbsps vegetable oil
- 1 clove garlic, crushed
- 1 stick of lemongrass (chop the inner stalk)
- 400g chicken breast, thinly sliced
- 1 small bunch of coriander, chopped
- 2 limes
- 2tbsps olive oil
- 1tbsp sweet chilli sauce

Method
Mix together the lettuce, cucumber, carrots and bean sprouts into a salad, and then divide between 4 individual plates. Heat the vegetable oil in a large frying pan or wok and gently cook the garlic and lemongrass for about 30 seconds, stirring so it doesn't burn. Turn up the heat to high, add the chicken and fry for 1-2 minutes, stirring constantly, until it has cooked through. Remove the meat from the pan and divide it between the plates of salad. Squeeze about 2 tablespoons of juice from the limes and add to the pan in which you cooked the chicken, together with the coriander, olive oil and chilli sauce. Stir for 1 minute, so it all heats through and comes together, season to taste, and then pour it over the chicken and salad as a dressing.

cals 260 | fat 12g | sat fat 3g | protein 28g

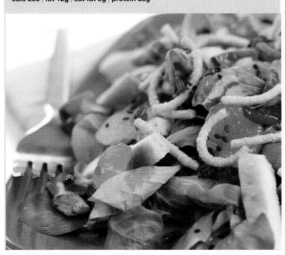

153

APPLE

DINNER

■ Vegetable soup (serves 4)

Ingredients
- 50g butter
- 2tbsps olive oil
- 1 medium leek, thinly sliced
- 1 medium carrot, peeled and diced
- 1 small potato, peeled and diced
- 1 stick of celery, thinly sliced
- 1 medium onion, diced
- 2 pinches of dried thyme
- 2tbsps plain flour
- 700ml vegetable or chicken stock
- 300ml milk
- 1 small head of broccoli, trimmed into small florets

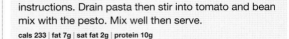

Method
Heat the butter and oil in a saucepan and gently sweat all the vegetables (except the broccoli) with the thyme for about 10 minutes, stirring every now and again, until softened, but not coloured. Add the flour to the pan and stir for 1 minute, then add the stock. Bring to the boil, stirring, and cook until thick, then add the milk. Season well and simmer for 10 minutes. Add the broccoli florets and continue cooking for another 5 minutes or until the broccoli is just done but still crunchy.

cals 374 | fat 9g | sat fat 4g | protein 12g

■ Easy pasta, beans and tomato (serves 4)

Ingredients
- 1tbsp olive oil
- 1 onion, finely chopped
- 1 large apple, cored and chopped
- 400g tin chopped tomatoes with garlic and herbs
- 300ml passata
- 290g tin borlotti beans, drained and rinsed
- 3tbsps red pesto
- 300g pasta shapes

Method
Heat oil in a pan and gently fry the onion for 3 minutes. Stir in the apple and cook for 2-3 minutes until both have softened. Stir in the tomatoes, passata and beans. Bring to the boil then simmer gently for 10 minutes. Meanwhile cook the pasta according to packet instructions. Drain pasta then stir into tomato and bean mix with the pesto. Mix well then serve.

cals 233 | fat 7g | sat fat 2g | protein 10g

■ Stir-fried prawns and red pepper (serves 2)

Ingredients
- 3tbsps groundnut or sunflower oil
- 2 garlic cloves, sliced thinly
- 1 small red pepper, deseeded and thinly sliced
- 200g raw peeled prawns, defrosted and patted dry
- 2tbsps soy sauce or Thai fish sauce
- 100g baby spinach leaves

Method
Heat a wok, add 2 tablespoons of oil and the garlic. Stir-fry until just golden, then spoon on to kitchen paper to drain. Add the pepper and stir-fry for 1 minute until slightly softened, then spoon out and set aside. Add the remaining tablespoon of oil. Heat, then toss in the prawns and stir-fry for 2-3 minutes until cooked and pink. Add the soy or fish sauce. Add the spinach and stir-fry until it begins to wilt. Return the peppers and garlic to the wok to heat through, mix well and serve.

cals 269 | fat 18g | sat fat 3g | protein 21g

■ Chicken burgers with lemon and mint (serves 4)

Ingredients
- 450g minced chicken or turkey
- ½ a small onion, grated
- Zest and juice of 1 lemon
- 1 garlic clove, finely chopped
- 3tbsps fresh mint, chopped
- Pinch of dried chilli flakes
- 1 beaten egg white

Method
Combine all the ingredients in a large bowl and mix thoroughly. Shape the mixture into 8 burgers about 2cm thick. Cover and leave in fridge for at least an hour to firm up, or they will fall apart during cooking. Heat a griddle or frying pan and cook the burgers for 4-5 minutes on each side. Serve them with a mixed salad and some low-fat mayonnaise.

cals 180 | fat 2.9g | sat fat 0.8g | protein 29.5g

154

DINNER

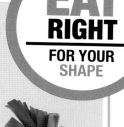

■ Broccoli and tuna frittata (serves 4)

Ingredients
- 200g broccoli florets
- 6 eggs
- 3tbsps snipped fresh chives
- 1tbsp olive oil
- 15g butter
- 418g tin of tuna in water, drained and flaked
- 198g tin of sweetcorn, drained
- 25g Parmesan cheese, grated

Method
Blanch the broccoli in lightly salted water for about 4 minutes. Beat the eggs with the chives and season. Heat the oil and butter in a large frying pan and pour in the egg mixture. Scatter over the broccoli, tuna and sweetcorn and, using a flat knife, pull the sides of the egg mixture in a little to allow the uncooked egg to set. Cook until the underside is golden and the top is almost set. Sprinkle with Parmesan and place under the grill for about 2-3 minutes until bubbling and golden. Serve cut into quarters, with a tomato or green salad.

cals 402 | fat 24g | sat fat 8g | protein 36.5g

■ Easy chicken kebabs (serves 4)

Ingredients
- 3 garlic cloves, roughly chopped
- 1 inch fresh ginger, roughly chopped
- 1 orange, grated zest and juice
- 3 spring onions, roughly chopped
- 2tbsps honey
- 1tbsp light soy sauce
- 2tbsps olive oil
- 4 skinless chicken breast fillets, cut into cubes
- 20 cherry tomatoes
- 2 large red peppers, each cut into 10 pieces

Method
Chop the garlic, ginger, orange zest and spring onions to a paste in a food processor. Then add the honey, orange juice, soy sauce and oil, and blend again. Pour the mixture over the chicken chunks and leave to marinate for at least 1 hour, but ideally overnight. Thread the chicken, tomatoes, and peppers on to wooden skewers, then cook on a hot griddle pan for 7-8 minutes each side or until the meat is thoroughly cooked and golden, turning frequently and basting with the marinade from time to time. Serve with a salad.

cals 110 | fat 9g | sat fat 2g | protein 8g

■ Tasty beef bake (serves 4)

Ingredients
- 2tbsps olive oil
- 1 onion, 1 carrot, 1 leek, 2 celery sticks – all diced
- 2 garlic cloves, chopped
- 75g mushrooms, sliced
- 500g braising steak, cubed
- 2tbsps plain flour
- 3 sprigs of thyme
- 750ml beef stock
- 2tbsps tomato purée
- 1 dash of Worcestershire sauce

Method
Heat 1 tablespoon of olive oil in a large pan then add the onion, carrot, leek, celery and garlic, and cook gently for 5 minutes without browning. Add the mushrooms and cook for a further 5 minutes, then remove everything from the pan and set aside. Heat a little more olive oil in the pan, add the beef and brown all over. Stir the flour in well. Return the veg to the pan and add the thyme, stock, purée and a dash of Worcestershire sauce. Season and mix well. Bring to a gentle simmer and cook, covered, for 1½ hours until tender, stirring occasionally. Serve with steamed broccoli and green beans.

cals 298 | fat 13g | sat fat 4g | protein 29.8g

■ Cod fillets with tomatoes and black olives (serves 4)

Ingredients
- 175g black olives in olive oil, stones removed
- 1 large onion, roughly chopped
- 400g tin chopped tomatoes
- 4 boneless cod fillets
- 1tbsp fresh flat-leaf parsley, chopped

Method
Preheat the oven to 180°C/350°/Gas Mark 4. Heat 1 tablespoon of the oil from the olives in an ovenproof pan. Add the onion and stir well, leave to cook for a minute or two, and then give the pan a good stir. Add the tomatoes and seasoning. Bring to the boil then add the olives. Put the fish, skin-side down, on to the sauce and drizzle over a splash more oil from the olive jar. Bake in the hot oven, uncovered, for 15 minutes. Sprinkle with the chopped parsley and serve.

cals 223 | fat 6g | sat fat 1g | protein 34g

155

PEAR

Pear-shaped physiques tend to crave sweet, creamy or starchy foods. They should opt for complex carbs like fresh fruit, wholegrain cereals, oats, Basmati rice and vegetables (except potatoes when made into chips or buttery mash). They should also eat plenty of protein including fish, lean meat and eggs, and avoid consuming saturated fats in the form of dairy products and fatty cuts of meat.

BREAKFAST

■ Fruit, yoghurt and toasted pumpkin seeds
Cut up 3 of your favourite fruits (such as an apple, a pear and a mango) and mix with 3tbsps of natural yoghurt. Sprinkle with some toasted pumpkin seeds.
cals 225 | fat 2.5g | sat fat 0.5g | protein 10g

■ Scrambled eggs on toast
Scramble 2 eggs with a dash of skimmed milk and add seasoning to taste. Spoon on to 1 slice of wholemeal toast and serve with 1 tomato, cut in half and grilled.
cals 324 | fat 3.8g | sat fat 1.6g | protein 18.8g

■ Cereal with fruit
Mix together 40g of bran flakes or All Bran with a chopped apple, a sliced banana and 125ml of semi-skimmed milk.
cals 265 | fat 3.5g | sat fat 1.5g | protein 8.5g

■ Porridge and yoghurt
Make a bowl of porridge in the microwave or on the hob with 40g of oats and semi-skimmed milk, according to packet instructions. Serve with 1tbsp of natural yoghurt in the middle.
cals 248 | fat 4.7g | sat fat 0.7g | protein 5.9g

■ Grilled bacon and poached egg on toast
Grill 2 rashers of back bacon and poach an egg. Serve on top of 1 slice of wholemeal toast with Flora Light.
cals 615 | fat 42.1g | sat fat 17.8g | protein 35.9g

■ Muesli with grated apple
A bowl of sugar-free muesli (50g) served with 1 peeled, grated apple and 125ml of semi-skimmed milk.
cals 350 | fat 5g | sat fat 1.5g | protein 10g

■ Mushrooms on toast
Heat 1tbsp of olive oil in a pan and quickly fry 50-60g thickly sliced mushrooms. Serve on 1 slice of wholemeal toast with Flora Light spread.
cals 255 | fat 16.3g | sat fat 2.8g | protein 5.6g

■ Tomatoes on toast
Heat 1 small tin of whole tomatoes, season and serve on 1 slice of wholemeal toast.
cals 145 | fat 1.3g | sat fat 0.8g | protein 3.2g

■ Breakfast fruit smoothie
Put 250ml of semi-skimmed milk, 60g of natural yoghurt, 125g of strawberries, the seeds of 2 passion fruits and 2tsps of honey into a blender. Process until smooth and drink straight away.
cals 205 | fat 4.8g | sat fat 3g | protein 6.5g

■ Cooked breakfast
For a special weekend treat, grill 1 lean sausage, 1 rasher of bacon, 1 large flat mushroom and 1 tomato, cut in half. Serve with 1 poached egg and 1 slice of wholemeal toast spread with Flora Light.
cals 517 | fat 25g | sat fat 12.3g | protein 21.7g

■ Shredded Wheat
A healthy cereal without any calorific nuts, honey or sugar coating! Simply serve 45g in a bowl with 125ml of semi-skimmed milk.
cals 210 | fat 3g | sat fat 1.5g | protein 9.5g

■ Boiled egg and soldiers
1 boiled egg and 1 slice of wholemeal toast with Flora Light spread, cut into fingers.
cals 220 | fat 8.6g | sat fat 2.3g | protein 11.1g

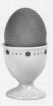

■ Toast and peanut butter
1 slice of wholemeal toast with peanut butter, served with 1 glass of orange juice.
cals 215 | fat 10.3g | sat fat 2.8g | protein 8.6g

■ Baked beans on toast
Reduced-sugar baked beans are a great source of fibre and protein. Serve 1 small can on 1 slice brown toast.
cals 210 | fat 1.3g | sat fat 0.8g | protein 12.2g

LUNCH

■ Crudités, houmous and pitta bread
Serve 1 small tub of low-fat houmous with 1 small warm wholemeal pitta bread cut into fingers. Add a few crudités, such as some raw carrot sticks, raw cauliflower florets and a red pepper, cut into strips.
cals 295 | fat 12g | sat fat 0g | protein 5.3g

■ Lentil soup
Buy a good quality lentil soup (check food label for fat content), or ideally make your own (see recipe on page 161). Serve with a wholemeal roll.
cals 238 | fat 7g | sat fat 1g | protein 11g

■ Chicken salad tortilla wrap
Warm 1 wholemeal tortilla wrap and fill with 3-4 slices cooked chicken, 1 handful of shredded lettuce, 1 chopped tomato and 1tbsp of low-fat mayonnaise.
cals 242 | fat 3.1g | sat fat 1.7g | protein 0g

■ Jacket potato with baked beans
Bake or microwave a small jacket potato and top with 1 small tin of baked beans. Ideally opt for reduced-sugar and reduced-salt versions of the beans.
cals 340 | fat 0.7g | sat fat 0g | protein 11g

■ Chicken and salad roll
Choose a normal-size wholemeal roll (rather than a huge bap) and fill with lean, roast chicken and salad of your choice. Spread the top half of the roll with a little low-fat mayonnaise.
cals 275 | fat 5g | sat fat 1.5g | protein 13.3g

■ Ham, lettuce and mustard sandwich
Make a sandwich from 2 slices of good quality, lean ham, some salad leaves and 2 pieces of thinly sliced wholemeal bread. Spread the bread with a thin layer of mustard rather than butter.
cals 290 | fat 5.1g | sat fat 2.1g | protein 21.2g

■ Cheese omelette and green salad
Make an omelette with 2 eggs and 1tsp of Flora Light in a frying pan. While cooking, sprinkle with 1tbsp of grated Cheddar cheese. Serve with a green salad.
cals 396 | fat 33g | sat fat 14g | protein 24g

■ Sardines and tomatoes on toast
Slice 1 large tomato and pan-fry gently in a little olive oil. When softened, add 3 sardine fillets from a tin to warm through. Place the cooked tomatoes and the hot sardines on a slice of wholemeal toast.
cals 257 | fat 8.6g | sat fat 3.3g | protein 21.2g

■ Omelette
Whisk 2 eggs in a bowl, put 1 small tablespoon of Flora Light in an omelette pan and heat gently. Pour in the egg mixture and let the heat set the egg. Top the egg with 1 thinly sliced mushroom, 1 thinly sliced tomato and 1tbsp of grated Cheddar. Finish off the cooking under a hot grill, until the omelette is golden on top.
cals 398 | fat 35g | sat fat 16g | protein 27.2g

■ Warmed pitta bread filled with ham salad
Fill 1 warm pitta bread with 2 slices of lean ham, 1 thinly sliced tomato, some shredded lettuce and 1tbsp of low-fat mayonnaise.
cals 255 | fat 7g | sat fat 1g | protein 17.5g

■ Grilled gammon and poached eggs
Grill some lean gammon for 3-4 minutes on each side and serve with 2 poached eggs.
cals 387 | fat 24.8g | sat fat 6.5g | protein 37.5g

■ Bagel with reduced-fat cream cheese
Split a bagel (toasted if preferred) in half and spread with a little low-fat cream cheese.
cals 280 | fat 7.5g | sat fat 3.5g | protein 9.5g

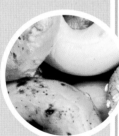

■ Tuna and egg salad
Make a mixed salad with chopped lettuce, 6 cherry tomatoes, cut in half, a few slices of cucumber and 6 olives. Drizzle with a little olive oil and top with 1 hard-boiled egg, cut into quarters, and 1 small tin of flaked tuna (in water).
cals 245 | fat 8.5g | sat fat 2.3g | protein 39.5g

■ Ryvita crackers with cottage cheese, celery and grapes
Top 2 Ryvitas, or other low-fat crispbreads, with 1 small pot of cottage cheese. Serve with 2-3 sticks of celery and a small bunch of grapes.
cals 115 | fat 2.5g | sat fat 1g | protein 8g

157

PEAR

DINNER

■ Spicy chicken fajitas (serves 4)
Ingredients
- 3 skinless chicken breasts
- 2tbsps Cajun spice mix
- 3tbsps olive oil
- Juice of 1 lime
- 8 soft wholemeal tortillas
- 1 pack baby leaf salad
- 8tbsps low-fat mayonnaise

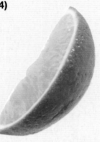

Method
Cut the chicken breasts lengthways into long strips and toss in the Cajun spice mix. Heat the olive oil in a large frying pan and stir-fry the coated chicken for around 6 minutes until cooked right through. Remove from the heat and sprinkle the chicken with lime juice. Warm some wholemeal tortillas and fill each with salad leaves, chicken strips, pan juices and mayonnaise. Roll up loosely and serve.

cals 509 | fat 11g | sat fat 2g | protein 35.5g

■ Creamy vegetable risotto (serves 4)
Ingredients
- 1L vegetable stock
- 100g asparagus, cut in half
- 100g baby carrots, cut in half lengthways
- 200g peas
- 500g broad beans
- 2tbsps olive oil
- 2 baby leeks, thinly sliced
- 300g risotto rice
- 1tbsp pesto
- 25g pine nuts, toasted

Method
Bring the vegetable stock to the boil in a large saucepan then reduce the heat. Add the asparagus, baby carrots, peas and broad beans. Simmer for 4-5 minutes until tender. Remove the veg with a slotted spoon and set aside. Keep the stock simmering. Meanwhile, heat the oil in a large frying pan and add the leeks. Stir-fry for 2 minutes, then stir in the rice.

Add 2-3 tablespoons of the hot stock and cook gently, stirring until the liquid is absorbed. Continue adding the stock, a little at a time, until the mixture has a 'soupy' texture and the rice is tender. This will take about 20 minutes. Stir in the pesto and season to taste. Gently stir in the vegetables that were put aside previously and heat through. Serve with toasted pine nuts scattered over the top.

cals 524 | fat 16g | sat fat 2g | protein 20g

■ Quick Thai chicken curry (serves 4)
Ingredients
- 400ml reduced-fat coconut milk
- 200ml chicken stock
- 2tbsps Thai green curry paste
- 4 skinless chicken breasts, cut into thin strips
- 350g new potatoes, cleaned and cut into chunks
- 6 spring onions, sliced diagonally
- 125g peas
- 2tbsps lime juice
- 1 red pepper, sliced
- 4tbsps fresh coriander, chopped

Method
Put the coconut milk, stock and Thai curry paste in a wok, stir together then heat until bubbling. Stir in the chicken and potatoes then bring back to the boil. Reduce the heat and simmer, uncovered, for about 15 minutes until the chicken and potatoes are just tender. Stir in the spring onions, lime juice, peas and red pepper and simmer for a further 4-5 minutes until everything is warmed through. Finally, stir in the coriander and season to taste.

cals 372 | fat 13g | sat fat 1g | protein 41g

158

DINNER

■ Broccoli and salmon frittata (serves 4)

Ingredients
- 200g broccoli florets
- 6 eggs
- 3tbsps snipped fresh chives
- 1tbsp olive oil
- 15g butter
- 2 tins (212g each) of red salmon, drained and flaked
- 198g tin sweetcorn, drained
- 25g Parmesan cheese, grated

Method
Blanch the broccoli in lightly salted water for about 4 minutes then drain well and set aside. Beat the eggs with the chives and season with freshly ground black pepper. Heat the oil and butter in a large ovenproof frying pan and pour in the eggs. Scatter over the broccoli, salmon and sweetcorn, stirring lightly to evenly distribute it all. Using a flat knife, pull the sides of the egg mixture in a little to allow the uncooked egg to set, and leave until the underside is golden and the top is almost set. Sprinkle with Parmesan and place under a hot grill for about 2-3 minutes until bubbling and golden (remember the frying pan handle will be hot). Serve cut into quarters, with a tomato or green salad.

cals 402 | fat 24g | sat fat 8g | protein 36.5g

■ Chicken and chorizo casserole (serves 4)

Ingredients
- 2tbsps olive oil
- 2 onions, chopped
- 2 garlic cloves, crushed
- 1tbsp fresh rosemary
- 40g chorizo sausage, skinned and diced
- 2 red peppers, deseeded and chopped
- 400g tin chopped tomatoes
- 3tbsps white wine
- 4 skinless chicken breasts
- 50g black or green olives, stoned

Method
Heat the oil in a casserole dish, add the onions, garlic and rosemary, and cook gently for about 15 minutes until soft and golden. Add the chorizo sausage and red peppers and cook over a moderate heat for a couple of minutes, then add the tinned tomatoes and wine. Season with freshly ground black pepper, stirring well, and bring to a simmer. Add the chicken and stir to coat with the sauce. Bring to the boil then reduce the heat to a simmer. Cover and cook for 30 minutes until the chicken is tender and cooked through. Just before serving, stir in the olives then check the seasoning and adjust if necessary.

cals 293 | fat 11g | sat fat 2g | protein 32g

■ Tomato and prawn pasta (serves 4)

Ingredients
- 250g pasta
- 2 red peppers, deseeded and cut into wide strips
- 1tbsp olive oil
- 16 raw tiger prawns
- 125ml tomato passata
- 2tbsps dry sherry (Fino or Manzanilla)
- 2tbsps fresh coriander

Method
Cook the pasta according to packet instructions. Heat a griddle pan and cook the pepper strips for about 3 minutes on each side until lightly charred. Remove from the heat and transfer to a bowl. Stir in the olive oil and cover. Quickly cook the prawns on the hot griddle for about 1 minute until pink, then add to the peppers. Gently heat the passata and sherry in a large saucepan, then add the cooked pasta with the peppers, prawns and chopped coriander. Toss together and serve.

cals 328 | fat 4g | sat fat 0.5g | protein 16g

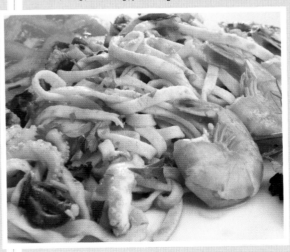

159

PEAR

DINNER

■ Roasted salmon (serves 4)
Ingredients
- 500g potatoes, peeled and sliced
- 1 aubergine, thickly sliced
- 4 large tomatoes, sliced
- 4 anchovies, drained, rinsed and finely chopped
- 2tbsps olive oil
- 1tbsp capers, chopped
- 4 salmon steaks
- 5tbsps low-fat mayonnaise
- Grated zest and juice of ½ lemon

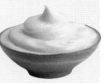

Method
Preheat oven to 200°C/390°F/Gas Mark 6. Cook the potatoes in boiling water for about 8 minutes until just tender, then drain. Arrange the potato, aubergine and tomato slices in overlapping rings in a large, lightly oiled roasting tin. In a small bowl, combine the anchovies, oil and capers and season with freshly ground black pepper. Pour this mixture over the vegetables. Cover and bake in the oven for 20 minutes. Arrange the salmon steaks on top of the vegetables, re-cover them and cook for 10 minutes. Uncover the tin and cook for a further 10 minutes. Meanwhile, in a small bowl, mix the mayonnaise with the lemon juice and zest, and serve with the salmon and the vegetables.
cals 502 | fat 28g | sat fat 5g | protein 35g

■ Broccoli and cauliflower gratin (serves 4)
Ingredients
- 1 large cauliflower
- 500g broccoli
- 3 spring onions, trimmed and sliced
- 25g cornflour
- 550ml semi-skimmed milk
- 75g mature Cheddar or Gruyère cheese, grated
- 1 egg, beaten
- 100g fresh breadcrumbs
- 25g walnut pieces

Method
Preheat oven to 190°C/370°F/Gas Mark 5. Trim the cauliflower, and cut both the cauliflower and broccoli into florets. Blanch for 1 minute in a large saucepan, then drain. Put the spring onions into the saucepan, and mix the cornflour with a little of the milk to make a smooth paste. Add the rest of the milk to the onions and bring to the boil. Stir half the hot milk into the cornflour mixture, then pour the mixture into the pan. Bring to the boil, stirring frequently, until you have a smooth sauce. Remove the sauce from the heat and stir in the cheese, beaten egg and half the breadcrumbs. Stir in the broccoli and cauliflower, and season to taste. Transfer all of this to an ovenproof baking dish, scatter over the rest of the breadcrumbs and the walnuts and bake for 20 minutes until golden.
cals 373 | fat 18g | sat fat 7g | protein 25g

■ Thai beef salad (serves 4)
Ingredients
- 350g lettuce leaves, shredded
- 175g cucumber, diced
- 2 carrots, peeled and grated
- 115g bean sprouts
- 4tbsps olive oil
- 1 clove of garlic, crushed
- 1 stick lemongrass (chop inner stalk)
- 500g lean steak, sliced
- 2 limes
- Small bunch coriander, chopped
- 1tbsp sweet chilli sauce

Method
Arrange the lettuce, cucumber, carrots and bean sprouts on individual plates. Heat 2 tablespoons of olive oil in a wok and gently cook the garlic and lemongrass for about 30 seconds. Add the steak and fry over a high heat for 1-2 minutes, stirring constantly. Remove the steak from the pan and place on salad vegetables. Squeeze 2 tablespoons of juice from the limes and add to the pan with the coriander, remaining olive oil and chilli sauce. Stir for 1 minute then pour over the salad.
cals 272 | fat 14g | sat fat 4g | protein 29g

160

DINNER

■ Grilled trout with walnut dressing (serves 4)

Ingredients
- 2tsps olive oil
- 4 trout fillets
- ¼tsp paprika
- 10 walnut halves
- 125g rocket, watercress or mixed leaves
- 3-4 boiled new potatoes

For the dressing
- 1 shallot, finely chopped
- Few sprigs of dill, chopped
- 2tbsps sherry vinegar
- 6tbsps walnut oil

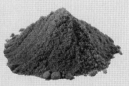

Method
Preheat the grill. Make the dressing by combining all the dressing ingredients in a small bowl and mixing well. Set aside. Grease the grill pan with half the oil and lay the trout fillets on top, skin-side down. Season with salt and paprika. Grill for 5-8 minutes, on one side only, until the flesh is opaque in the centre. While the trout is cooking, heat the remaining oil in a small frying pan and gently fry the walnuts, stirring constantly so that they colour but do not burn. Drain on kitchen paper then chop roughly. Arrange the salad leaves on individual plates. Lay a trout fillet on top. Stir the dressing to bring it together, spoon it over the top and scatter with nuts. Serve with the new potatoes.

cals 451 | fat 33g | sat fat 4g | protein 37g

■ Turkey burgers with lemon and mint (serves 4)

Ingredients
- 450g minced turkey
- ½ a small onion, grated
- Zest and juice of 1 lemon
- 1 garlic clove, finely chopped
- 3tbsps mint, chopped
- Pinch of dried chilli flakes
- 1 beaten egg white

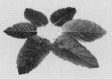

Method
In a bowl, combine all the ingredients, mix thoroughly and season. Shape the mixture into 8 burgers about 2cm thick. Cover and leave in the fridge for at least 1 hour to firm up, or they will fall apart when you cook them. Heat a griddle or frying pan until hot and cook the burgers for 4-5 minutes on each side. Serve with a mixed salad and low-fat mayonnaise.

cals 180 | fat 2.9g | sat fat 0.8g | protein 29.5g

■ Spicy lentil and carrot soup

Ingredients
- 2tsps cumin seeds
- 1 pinch chilli flakes
- 2tbsps olive oil
- 600g carrots, diced
- 140g split red lentils
- 1L hot vegetable stock
- 125ml milk

Method
Heat a large saucepan and dry-fry the cumin seeds and chilli flakes for 1 minute, or until they start to jump around the pan, releasing their aromas. Scoop out about half of the seeds with a spoon and set aside. Carefully add the oil, carrot, lentils, stock and milk to the pan and bring to the boil. Simmer for 15 minutes or until the lentils have swollen and softened. Whizz the soup with a blender until smooth (or leave it chunky if you prefer). Add the remaining spices and season.

cals 238 | fat 7g | sat fat 1g | protein 11g

■ Sausage and butter bean casserole (serves 4)

Ingredients
- 6 lean sausages
- 1tbsp olive oil
- 6 slices of streaky bacon, chopped
- 1 large leek, sliced
- 1 garlic clove, sliced
- 125ml of white wine
- 200ml chicken stock
- 1 pinch of chilli flakes
- 2 x 400g tins of butter beans, drained and rinsed
- 1 small bunch of parsley, roughly chopped

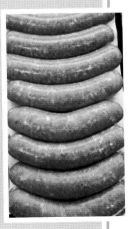

Method
Brown the sausages in a little oil, and slice into chunks. Brown the bacon in the same pan, then add the leek and garlic, and cook till softened. Return the sausages to the pan with the wine, stock, chilli flakes and butter beans. Simmer for 10-15 minutes until the sausages are cooked through. Top with the parsley.

cals 474 | fat 28.6g | sat fat 9g | protein 26g

161

Top 10 simple food tricks

1. Swap the plates you eat off for smaller ones.

2. If you live with a man, don't eat the same quantities as him!

3. Eat off a blue plate as this is said to suppress your appetite.

4. Don't cut out dairy products – studies show eating dairy aids weight-loss.

5. Drink at least two litres of water a day – it boosts your metabolism, plus many people mistake thirst for hunger.

6. Add protein to every meal, it will keep you fuller for longer.

7. Never skip breakfast: this causes your body to store fat.

8. Eat little and often to avoid excess calories being stored as bodyfat.

9. Don't go food shopping when you're hungry as you'll opt for high-sugar foods that contain 'empty' calories.

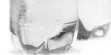

10. Add spices like cinnamon, turmeric and chilli to your meals to boost your metabolism.

162